Understanding Your Moods
When You're Expecting

Understanding Your Moods
When You're Expecting

Emotions,
Mental Health,
and Happiness —
Before, During,
and After
Pregnancy

LUCY J. PURYEAR, M.D.

HOUGHTON MIFFLIN COMPANY

BOSTON • NEW YORK

2007

Visit our Web site: www.houghtonmifflinbooks.com.

Library of Congress Cataloging-in-Publication Data

Puryear, Lucy J.
Understanding your moods when you're expecting : emotions,
mental health, and happiness — before, during, and after
pregnancy / Lucy J. Puryear.
p. cm.
Includes index.
ISBN: 978-0-547-05362-2
ISBN-10: 0-618-34107-2
1. Pregnancy — Popular works. 2. Pregnancy — Psychological
aspects. 3. Childbirth — Popular works. 4. Child care —
Popular works. I. Title.
RG525.P87 2007 618.2 — dc22 2006035606

Printed in the United States of America

Book design by Victoria Hartman

MP 10 9 8 7 6 5 4 3 2 1

To my mother, MARTHA,
and her mother, GLADYS,
and to my daughters,
KATIE and MAGGIE,
and their daughters

Contents

Acknowledgments

It has taken me more than four years to give birth to this book. When I started this project, I had no idea how difficult it was to bring a book to completion. It takes a female elephant twenty-two months to deliver a baby; I could have had two by now.

I know I would not be celebrating the arrival of this book without the help, support, and patience of numerous people.

I would like to thank the three women who were midwives to me and have been my own personal support group: Joy Harris, my literary agent, who immediately said yes and has taken care of me from day one; Deanne Urmy of Houghton Mifflin, who had a vision of what this book could be and who believed in it and understood it from the beginning; and the indefatigable and always positive Jane Isay, who took me in during the storm and encouraged me to get this book finished. Jane's hand and words are seen throughout, and I am also happy to count her as a new friend.

Thanks to my writer friends, Marcy McKay and Suzy Spencer, who welcomed me into the club and gave wonderful support and advice. Thanks also to Glenn Cambor, M.D., and Lauren Marangell, M.D., who read an early draft and gave me clear direction.

I am grateful for my children, Katie, Mason, Will, and Maggie, who have been unflaggingly excited and still tell all their friends and anyone else who will listen that their mom is writing a book. They look at me with eyes that show me my best self.

This book would not be what it is without the many women and their families who have trusted me to help them through difficult times and have allowed me to share their joys and successes. Although the stories in this book do not represent real patients of mine, their voices can be heard throughout.

And thanks to Jamie, who stands beside me and smiles.

Understanding Your Moods
When You're Expecting

Introduction

Growing up as a young girl in Baltimore in the sixties and seventies, I watched in fascination as women fought for equal rights. But I didn't fully understand why they had to fight for them. As the firstborn child of a man who wanted a son, I was treated like one. My father claims I knew the names of all the positions on a football team by the time I was two. I was allowed to do anything the boys did. My father taught me how to throw an almost perfect spiral and how to shoot a rifle and hunt dove in the Rio Grande Valley. I read the books he'd read as a boy and couldn't imagine that girls could be treated differently than boys.

From watching television, I knew about Gloria Steinem, Billie Jean King, and the campaign for the Equal Rights Amendment. I wasn't old enough to have a bra to burn, but I would have burned it if I had been. I was determined not to let the fact that I had been born female stop me, and my parents confirmed that I could do anything I wanted to do. A desire was born in me to accomplish something that made a difference.

As a college student, I became involved in women's health issues and thought about becoming a midwife or an obstetrician. But as I watched the doctors working in the clinic where I volunteered, I became disillusioned with the way some of them dealt with their female patients. These doctors often treated the women's physical symptoms but ignored or trivialized their emotional complaints. When at age twenty-five I complained to my own gynecologist about having premenstrual mood swings, he literally patted me on the head and with a patronizing smile said, "Lots of women have that, honey. Don't worry about it."

I was embarrassed and furious at the same time. I felt like an overly emotional little girl and angry that my complaint hadn't been taken seriously. At that moment, I decided that I would go to medical school and become a different kind of doctor. I would be a physician who listened and treated women with respect. I imagined myself as an obstetrician who sat by women's sides as they delivered their babies, listened to their stories, and educated them about their bodies.

I began medical school and was soon confronted with the limitations of the health care system. I realized how difficult it would be to practice obstetrics in the way I'd fantasized. There doesn't seem to be enough time in the day for doctors to see as many patients as necessary to make a living and also to have a personal life outside of work. The legal climate forces physicians to practice defensive medicine, performing procedures that may not be necessary. New technology often causes doctors to treat lab results or monitors instead of patients.

The few female obstetric residents I knew were subtly conditioned to act like their male counterparts — tough and efficient — to be respected. There was no handholding or staying with a woman while she labored. It was often the nurses who delivered the baby. The doctor's arrival was carefully timed to appear when the baby was almost born and there was not much left to do but cut an episiotomy and sew it up. It was not that the doctors were lazy or didn't want to be there; it was just that they had too many women to care for, had too much paperwork, and were too sleep deprived.

In medical school, as I contemplated what the next step for me would be, I was torn. Delivering babies was fun. It is amazing to help a woman give birth through her struggles and her pain. I could watch the television show *Maternity Ward* for hours on end and never tire of seeing the mixture of relief and awe on the mother's face when her infant was finally delivered.

Being privileged to help guide babies into the world is an incredible feeling. But I had a young daughter and wanted more children. An ob-gyn residency is very difficult, and I knew life wouldn't get much better once I was finished. Many obstetricians stop delivering babies after several years due to malpractice insurance costs and the great demands the work makes on one's life. My concerns about whether I could be the kind of doctor that I wanted to be only grew.

Gradually, I realized that psychiatry was a field that could allow me to practice medicine in such a way that I could be fully attentive to the whole woman. As a resident in psychiatry, I couldn't wait to get up in the morning and go to the hospital. I looked forward to reading everything I could about psychiatric illness and its treatment. The patients were fascinating. Each day would bring a new story, a new tale of human strength in the face of suffering. I learned that all of us have pain in our lives and all of us have families that are less than perfect. As a general physician, I could treat pneumonia or diabetes and save someone's life. Yet as a psychiatrist, I could help people out of chaos in a way that allowed them and their families to live in the world with joy and hope.

During my psychiatry residency, I was asked to help teach ob-gyn residents about diagnosing and treating psychiatric illness. I began to work in the high-risk obstetrics clinic at Houston's Ben Taub General Hospital. There I saw pregnant women who had histories of psychiatric illness or had developed psychiatric symptoms during their pregnancies. It was my job to decide whether medication was necessary and if so which medication would be safest to use.

After several months as attending psychiatric resident in the high-risk clinic, the ob-gyn residents began to seek me out to ask questions about their patients. They became more interested in evaluating and treating their patients for emotional symptoms. Women from outlying community clinics began to be referred to Ben Taub for the specialized treatment we were offering. I was increasingly asked to give lectures to other health care providers about psychiatric illness during pregnancy. My future now seemed clear to me.

I realized that there was a huge hole in the mental health care available to pregnant women. Many women wouldn't ask for help out of fear and shame. Many were told they couldn't get treatment while they were pregnant. They were told that because they had depression, anxiety, or bipolar disorder, they shouldn't have children. They also were told that they were at risk of losing custody of their children if they remained mentally ill. And when a woman with a psychiatric diagnosis became pregnant, I was not infrequently asked to decide whether the state should take the infant away after delivery.

This presented a terrible challenge. I was being asked to decide whether a mother was going to be too sick to care for her baby and to evaluate whether the baby would be better off in what I knew was a woefully inadequate foster care system. Unless I could prove otherwise, it was assumed that a woman who had a psychiatric illness could not be a good mother. The women themselves faced a dilemma: they were being told on the one hand that psychiatric medication was not an option during pregnancy, but on the other hand that if they remained psychiatrically ill, they might not be able to care for their children and could even lose their right to parent.

This experience intensified my desire to advocate for women with psychiatric illness. People with mental illness make many of us uncomfortable and frightened. Historically, it was easier to lock mentally ill people up and ignore them. But all of us at some point in our lives will either have an emotional illness or know someone who does. One out of four women will develop a depressive illness at some time in her life. That could be you or me, your sister or your mother. And all of us have moments when we struggle with sadness or frustration or feel overwhelmed. Although we may not be diagnosed with an identifiable psychiatric disorder, we may often find life tumultuous and stressful.

After four years of residency, I joined the faculty at Baylor College of Medicine in Houston. I started a women's psychiatric clinic and began to teach psychiatry residents and medical students how to care for women of reproductive age. I knew that I had found my place — taking care of women who were struggling with mood symptoms during reproductive events in their lives. For me this is the perfect combination of obstetrics, gynecology, and psychiatry.

Some people call this specialty reproductive psychiatry. At the time I started my professional life, very few psychiatrists knew about the interplay between women's hormonal fluctuations and their moods and mental health. I became an expert in treating women with severe premenstrual syndrome (PMS), pregnancy and psychiatric illness, postpartum mood disorders, and depression during perimenopause.

Today there are more women asking for this specialized type of care than I could possibly see. Some of my patients come from very far away because there is no one in their area with the specialized knowledge to care for them during pregnancy or the postpartum period. Many women slip through the cracks. Many obstetricians and gynecologists are not trained to recognize the signs and symptoms of psychiatric disorders. They typically see a woman six weeks after she delivers her baby and then not again for a year.

Future doctors need to learn more about issues specific to women, not just regarding psychiatric symptoms but also other diseases as well. Heart disease is a good example. For years people believed that women did not have heart attacks. Now we know that the symptoms women experience during a heart attack are often very different from those that men complain of. Women die from heart attacks because of the failure of medical science to pay attention to their specific needs.

Unfortunately, women who have emotional problems during pregnancy or after the baby is born nearly always feel shame and guilt. This compounds the problem of getting the right help. They believe that if they are experiencing anything besides great joy, all the time, they are bad mothers. Women often don't talk with helpful seriousness about the baby blues or about how having a baby was harder than they expected. These aren't common topics during prenatal classes or at baby showers. Instead, we all talk about how excited we are and how cute those tiny clothes are. If a new mother has difficulty adjusting, she will more likely suffer in silence than seek help.

On the first day of my psychiatry class with the first-year medical students at Baylor College of Medicine, I ask, "How many here have asthma?" Five to ten students usually raise their hands. "How many have GI [gastrointestinal] reflux?" Another three to five. When I ask, "How many have mental illness?" stillness falls over the 168 students present. A few people may giggle. I rephrase my inquiry. "Okay, how many people in this room have a family member or know someone with mental illness?" Just about everyone's hand goes up. I never really expect anyone, in a room full of their peers, to fess up to having mental illness themselves, but the exercise dramatically makes my point. It is not socially acceptable to have a psychiatric disorder. It is particularly difficult to be a new mother who is feeling less than happy about having had a baby.

It is time to acknowledge how disabling psychiatric illness during pregnancy and the postpartum period can be for both women and their families and how proper recognition and treatment can change their lives for generations. It is also time to realize that being pregnant and having a baby is hard work both physically and psychologically. It is not always fun being a mother. Most mothers would never choose to give up the experience, but they all need support and understanding. Knowing what may lie ahead can bring women one step closer to knowing when they may need help. Early recognition and treatment of symptoms may prevent more serious problems from arising.

Many books discuss the joys and pitfalls of pregnancy. These books offer information about the physical symptoms a pregnant woman may experience and common remedies to alleviate heartburn, sleepless nights, and lower back pain. Methods of delivery are reviewed, and women are encouraged to choose the type of birth that fits their physical and emotional needs.

But very few of these books talk about women's emotional health before, during, and after pregnancy. Some give helpful information about postpartum depression and anxiety, but most women will turn to such books only after they've experienced distressing symptoms.

Understanding Your Moods When You're Expecting is an in-depth look at the spectrum of feelings that women may experience, from the normal to symptoms that are more problematic, for which professional help may be required. It is an attempt to focus on psychological health and to acknowledge that the emotional issues that arise during and after pregnancy are as important as the physical ones. Having a baby isn't just a physical experience; it's a profound emotional experience as well. This book provides essential information for women who are pregnant or wish to become pregnant and for their families.

The book explains options available to new mothers who are struggling with thoughts and feelings they did not expect. When are the feelings serious and medical help necessary? What medications can you take while you are pregnant and breastfeeding? When should you consider medication, and when are other treatments a better choice? Can psychotherapy help?

The book also contains information that will help keep women and their families whole and healthy during pregnancy, childbirth, and the postpartum period. It gives voice to the doubts and anxieties that every mother feels even while she is experiencing the joy of bringing a new life into the world. Talking about the emotional upheavals of pregnancy and childbirth can prevent women from suffering in silence and reduce the risk that women who need help may not get it.

Understanding Your Moods When You're Expecting discusses the normal emotional and psychological responses to pregnancy and childbirth. Most women do not suffer from a diagnosable psychiatric illness during or after pregnancy. Yet all women have good days and bad days. They may be confused about what they are feeling and not know whether their feelings are common and short-lived or more serious and longer-term.

Many of the women who come to see me say, "If only I'd

known what to expect. Why didn't anyone tell me how hard it could be?" If women and their families can be empowered to get the help they need, potential suffering and tragedy can be avoided. Many women experience mood changes in response to normal hormonal fluctuations. Until recently, little attention was paid to what causes those symptoms and how to respond to them effectively. It is important for women and their families, and for the physicians who treat women, to realize that the reproductive years are a time when women's mental health is linked to what is happening to them hormonally. In addition, women with postpartum mood disorders are at increased risk for a recurrence with subsequent pregnancies and around the time of menopause.

Being pregnant and giving birth is a time of great biological and physiological change. A woman is not only experiencing physical changes that can be overwhelming, but she is also trying to adapt to emotional and psychological changes as well. A mother is not created when her baby is born, but when she can wrap her mind around what it means to *her* to be a mother.

On the Way to Motherhood

In virtually all cultures, pregnant women are admired and protected. They are taken care of and allowed to be needy and demanding. The presence of an obviously pregnant woman still causes a man to give up his seat on the subway or bus. The pregnant woman is seen as protecting an important life inside her, and many hopes and fantasies are projected onto her protruding belly. We all smile at the thought of a pregnant woman craving mango sorbet in the middle of a December night. Her partner may even sigh indulgently, put on his overcoat and boots, and go out in search of it.

When you think of being pregnant, you are imagining yourself full of health and looking forward to feeling the baby move inside you. You can't wait for all the smiles and hugs of your friends and family when you tell them the good news. You may look forward to being the center of attention, nurtured and cared for. You dream of holding your newborn in your arms, dressing him or her in adorable blue or pink clothes, and smelling his or her sweet baby smell. But actually being a mother is a concept that is still foreign to you. Others have been there, but what will it be like for you? You may be frightened of the unknown, and you may try to hide those feelings in the face of everyone else's excitement.

Bringing a new being into the world is an amazing prospect, and some women enjoy every minute of pregnancy. Most women *wish* they felt good about everything, but they don't. Worries about competency, about relationships, and about how life is going to change are universal. The more a woman tries to suppress those feelings, the greater effect they will have on her moods. It turns out that ambivalence is not only a universal feeling, but it's also a good thing. Taking the time to consider your fears, worries, and even sorrows will help you to be less demanding of yourself and eventually more accepting of your baby as an individual and of yourself as a mother.

I Think I Want to Be Pregnant

When Carmen arrived for her regular therapy appointment and told me she was pregnant, I wasn't sure how to react. I knew that she and her husband hadn't planned on having any more children, and the look on her face was one of shock. I asked how she felt about being pregnant.

"Well, it's weird," she said. "You know I don't want any more kids, but when I saw the pink plus sign on the stick, I felt excited. Then it hit me, all that was involved with having another baby, and I started to cry. And then the stupidest thing is that a few days later, I started to have some bleeding, and I was upset I might miscarry. Then I stopped bleeding, and I was disappointed. I think I'm losing my mind." Carmen threw up her hands in frustration and laughed.

Carmen was able to express clearly the situation many women

are in when they first find out they're pregnant. Knowing you're going to have a baby is both exhilarating and terrifying. Having negative thoughts about being pregnant does not mean that you won't love your baby or that you'll be a bad mom. All it means is that you are having normal worries about the awesome responsibilities of being a parent. It is important to acknowledge those thoughts as part of the process of becoming a mother and to move forward.

※

I RAN INTO my friend Jeannie waiting in line at the local coffee shop. We are both really busy, and it's a treat to get to hang out with her for a few minutes trading gossip. Usually Jeannie could rattle off her order with confidence, but today she was stumbling — trying to order a decaf latte but unable to choose from the list of decaf varieties. Jeannie and I are both caffeine addicts and drink two or three cups of coffee a day. Why was she ordering decaf?

I looked at her with a big smile and raised an eyebrow. Jeannie returned my grin and nodded. Then her smile began to fade, and her eyes filled with tears. I moved through the line to give her a hug, and she began to cry.

"I'm thrilled," she said. "It's wonderful. Greg and I haven't been trying for very long, and I just found out." Then why was she crying? Because, like every other newly pregnant woman, she was overwhelmed. She was scared. If she didn't know how to order her latte, imagine what else she didn't know.

We sat down at a table and began to talk. Jeannie is a well-respected psychiatrist. She is one of the first names that come to mind if I need a referral for a family member or a good friend. It can take weeks to get an appointment with her because she is so good at what she does. At the age of thirty-five, she's been in practice for five years and has worked hard to build her reputation. Jeannie grew up in the Northwest, but she came to Texas for medical school and never left. She met Greg in school, and they have a strong marriage. He has a job in a group practice in town, and they are happy where they are.

It was a good time for them to have a baby. Jeannie was worried that she might have infertility issues at her age, but it all happened easily and quickly. Now that the reality of being pregnant was sinking in, however, Jeannie was scared. She was very close to her family and missed them all the time. Although she made several trips home each year, the news of her pregnancy made her miss her mother more than ever. "I worry she's not really going to know the baby," Jeannie said with a sigh. "I can't do this alone. I may have been to medical school, but I'm clueless about babies. I don't even know how to change a diaper — I'm the baby of the family." All of a sudden, this highly competent woman felt incompetent.

The mixed feelings Jeannie was having are not just normal; they're universal. Remember graduating from school? You received a diploma and were told that it conveyed to you all the rights and responsibilities of an education. At that moment, you realized that your world was changing radically. The day you had been waiting for had finally arrived, and you were embarking on a new life. But the butterflies in your stomach also signaled there was no going back. You were no longer a fun-loving student, but a full-blown adult expected to function in a very different way.

Getting pregnant is one of those graduation moments. The rights, joys, and pleasures of motherhood are enormous. There's nothing like loving a child and receiving his love in return. There's nothing as fascinating as watching him grow into a unique, complicated human being. That tiny person with his own personality and quirks is the best thing that ever happened to you.

But this morning, Jeannie was overwhelmed by the responsibilities of becoming a parent. And she had another worry. Greg comes from a huge, loud, in-your-face family that lived near enough to visit frequently. One of the things that had made Jeannie fall in love with Greg was his close connection to his family. There were lots of family barbecues and birthday celebrations, with kids falling all over each other. Everyone welcomed Jeannie with enthusiasm and teased her as if she were one of them.

But now she was worried that Greg's family would overwhelm her new, beginning family and that she'd get lost in the crowd. How would she survive the endless family gatherings feeling the way she did? What if the baby was fussy when they visited or didn't get along with the cousins? Although she was accustomed to the noise and chaos of Greg's family, she didn't know how a newborn would take to it.

This was a subject she would rather not discuss with Greg. After all, she knew that having a big family and being close to them was going to be terrific for their baby. Greg was looking forward to adding their kids to the group and couldn't wait to tell his parents there was another grandchild on the way. She didn't want to spoil the excitement for him. But Jeannie's family was small and more reserved, and this melding of family cultures was another concern in Jeannie's calculation of impending motherhood. All of a sudden, things that had been only nagging worries in the back of her mind were coming to the fore as potential realities that she had to deal with.

Pregnant women might feel better if they knew that recognizing and confronting all their feelings is excellent preparation for the ups and downs of motherhood. And talking honestly with friends, family, and other mothers is a way to put the negative (and positive) feelings in perspective so as not to feel so frightened and overwhelmed.

Take, for instance, Jeannie's worry about being so far from her mother. If she voiced those thoughts out loud, there could be ways to make her family feel less far away. Her mother could be having the same feelings but not want to intrude on Jeannie and Greg, or maybe she was afraid to make Jeannie feel sad. If they both acknowledged their concerns, they could start making plans to reduce the impact of the distance between them. Jeannie could send her mother pictures from her ultrasounds so that her mom could be part of the excitement. They could work on planning the nursery together and send each other pictures of cribs and fabrics via e-mail.

Now was the time for Jeannie to start thinking about having her mother come to stay for a while after the baby was born. Maybe she could afford a webcam, so that her mom could see the baby "live" for several minutes every day. It's not easy being thousands of miles away from your family, but Jeannie did have friends and colleagues in town who would support her when her family couldn't be there.

As for Greg's family, Jeannie may come to realize that they are loving enough to make room for a quiet mother and child. And learning to enjoy a little roughhousing is not a bad thing for a child. Jeannie may be surprised to find out that Greg feels the same way she does and that he may be willing to run some interference with his family, especially in the beginning.

Thinking about all the things that will change when you become a mother for the first time is scary. You can anticipate some things, but others will just happen without your ever having imagined them. Your feelings will be complicated and powerful. There will be joys and sorrows, excitement and disappointment. It is important to remember that your (and your family's) journey will not look like anyone else's. Your feelings, both good and bad, will make the experience of motherhood unique and wonderful, and sometimes frightening and frustrating. Remember that any negative feelings you may have when you are pregnant are not an indication of your value as a mother. But it is important to recognize, honor, and deal with those feelings. Throughout this chapter, you'll find stories about women beginning their journey to motherhood and how they have dealt with their natural, universal, and legitimate feelings.

Working Through Family Relationships

Pregnancy often raises issues that have been suppressed or put aside. For a woman, becoming a mother forces her to rethink her relationship with her own mother — to see herself as both the same as and different from the single most important woman in her life. Even with the best mother-daughter relationships, women reflect on what kind of mother they had and what kind of mother they are going to be. In the worst of these relationships, women's confidence in their ability to mother may be severely compromised. They may feel as if they shouldn't have children at all out of fear that they will be doomed to repeat the past.

❧

REBECCA CAME TO see me when she was pregnant with her first child. She was having tremendous anxiety and felt as if something was continuously stuck in her throat. Her obstetrician referred her to me after a thorough exam during which he could find no physical causes for her symptoms.

As a psychiatrist, I am very cautious about dismissing people's physical symptoms as purely psychological. Historically, people with psychiatric symptoms have received less than adequate medical evaluations. It is imperative that a doctor thoroughly evaluate all physical symptoms before deciding that they are psychological in origin. Even symptoms that are "all in your head" can be disabling.

Rebecca was having difficulty functioning and taking care of her usual responsibilities. She was afraid she would have trouble breathing while she was driving or shopping in the grocery store. She had slowly limited her interaction with the outside world, preferring to stay close to home in case she had another "attack." Her obstetrician had noted that she was very anxious about her pregnancy and called frequently to make sure everything she was feeling was normal. The pregnancy was going well, but she was worried about how she would cope with a small child and whether she would be able to return to work after she delivered.

I spent an hour with Rebecca taking a careful psychiatric and medical history. Eventually, I asked, "What about growing up in your family? Are your parents still living?"

"My mom and dad are still living, but they divorced when I was two. I lived with my mom until I was fifteen, and then I went to live with my father."

I wondered about the fairly unusual situation of a teenage girl living with her father rather than with her mother. "What was that about? Why did you go live with your dad?" I asked.

"Well, my mom and I didn't get along. We had a big fight, and she said if I didn't like it, I could go live with my father. I said okay and left. I didn't talk to her for about two years after that. She'd call occasionally but would hang up if my dad answered the phone. They hate each other."

"They still don't get along?"

"No. It's pretty bad. My dad wouldn't come to my high school graduation because my mom was going to be there. The only person who ended up coming was my grandmother. She has been there for me the whole time. She thinks both my mom and dad are pretty ridiculous."

Rebecca had an older sister who had a child. I wondered how the birth of her baby had gone. Often families will put aside their differences when there is a new baby in the family. "Tell me about your sister's delivery," I said. "How was it? Was your family there?"

"That was a disaster. Both my mom and dad showed up while she was in labor. And then her husband's parents were there, too. It was crazy. My mom and dad got in a big fight about which one of them had to leave, and the in-laws were trying to mediate. My sister's poor husband was trying to take care of her in the delivery room and settle things in the waiting room. I sat in the corner and tried to stay out of the way. Both my parents ended up leaving. I guess it was for the best."

I noticed that Rebecca seemed fairly matter-of-fact while telling these stories. I said, "I wonder why, since you are telling me something that must be very painful for you, you don't look sad."

"Well, I think I've just tried to put their feuding behind me. I decided I was going to move on with my life and not worry about it anymore. There's nothing I can really do about it anyway. That's just the way things are."

I said, "You know, I'm wondering if being pregnant hasn't

stirred up all the old feelings again, even though you believed you'd put them behind you. I think they're making themselves known through physical symptoms, and that's where your anxiety is coming from."

"But what's the point of being sad about my parents not getting along? They are not going to change."

"Maybe they will, and maybe they won't, but you're still being affected by your feelings about them," I said. "If we try to understand what those feelings are and to acknowledge them as real and valid, maybe they won't be so overwhelming, and you won't have to keep them a secret from yourself. It's not surprising that thinking about becoming a mother has stirred up feelings about your own parents."

I explained to Rebecca that an especially troubling experience doesn't really go away. A woman may not be thinking constantly about what happened to her as a child, but it still may be having an effect on her body through anxiety, headaches, high blood pressure, or stomach upset. Memories resurface under certain circumstances — in Rebecca's case, her pregnancy. Now the very powerful emotional experience of being pregnant was bringing up both memories from her past and the feelings they evoked. It was a double whammy.

Rebecca and I spent three more sessions talking about her family and the profound disappointment she felt that her parents couldn't get along for her sake. She had always imagined that her having children would bring them together again. Now that she was pregnant, she had to grieve the fact that that wasn't going to happen.

Rebecca and I were able to talk about things she might do to make the birth of her new baby as peaceful and memorable as possible. Her mother and father agreed that they would come one at a time, with a day separating their visits. Rebecca was able to tell them that if either one of them caused a scene, they would not be welcome. Feeling that she had a right to be in control of her own situation and having a plan made her much less anxious. When Rebecca started to feel panicky, she used relaxation techniques to reduce her anxiety. She was not going to let the old family dynamics control her any longer.

You don't need to have lived through such a bitter family struggle to be anxious about how your long-divorced parents are going to react to your new baby. Many people harbor a sense of guilt and responsibility over their parents' divorce. Of course that's wholly unrealistic, but it is a common response to the breakup of a family. Some people also hold on to the dream that their parents will come back together at some time in the future. At the time when you are thinking about creating a new family unit, the sense of loss — that you didn't have the kind of security you are now intent on creating — can be heightened. Dealing with that loss can help you reconsider your old feelings and perhaps even recognize them for what they are — the thoughts and dreams of childhood. For many men and women, becoming a parent marks an important transition between childhood fantasies and adult understanding.

❧

AMY LOST HER mother, Paige, one of my close friends, when she was in her twenties and just out of college. Paige died in a freak accident. Divorced when her two kids were small, she had supported them and furthered her own education without complaint. After she died, I tried to keep up with her kids as best I could. I was thrilled that Amy invited me and her mother's other close friends to her wedding. As we entered the sanctuary, we saw an empty seat in front that held a single red rose — a message to her mother that all was well. It was a beautiful wedding, a tribute to the bride and her mother.

Now Amy's career was booming, and she was happy in her marriage. When my friends and I heard the news that Amy was expecting, we were all excited. Of course, Paige would have been ecstatic. She would have gone maternity clothes shopping with Amy and helped her plan the nursery, making her laugh the whole time. When Amy told me about her pregnancy, the first words out of my mouth were, "Your mother would be happy," and then I saw the sadness in Amy's eyes.

Amy is a strong and determined young woman, and she is generally confident that things are going to continue to be just fine. But when we had lunch a couple of weeks after her big announcement, she bowed her head and said, "My mom was the best." I nodded in agreement and waited for her to continue.

"She was an amazing mother, sacrificing herself for me and Matt, and always there for us." Again I assented.

After a long pause, Amy asked, "How can I do it? I've never spent time with little kids. I've never even burped a baby." I didn't have an answer that would keep her from missing her mother.

The next time we got together, Amy sounded a bit more cheerful, but still not great. She wanted to talk about her mother's death. "I can't get her memorial service out of my head," she said. "It felt as if Mom were there, sitting beside me in the church."

Amy wanted her mother back, and for good reason. Becoming a mother is a powerful reminder of your relationship with your own mother. Women who are very close to their mothers have the great benefit of a loving presence at their side, but they still worry about how they will take on the formidable task of parenting when Mom isn't around. Even if your mother is alive, she may not be able to spend a lot of time with you because of distance or the demands of her own life. If this is the case, you may feel just as isolated as Amy did.

When a woman becomes pregnant, it's common for her (and her husband) to remember experiences from her own childhood. It's not unusual, in the early stages of pregnancy, to start considering what you want to re-create from your childhood and what you want to make sure absolutely does not happen to your own child. This review of your childhood and your parents' parenting skills is important, even if you experience feelings of loss or resentment. Such feelings might seem like diversions from the tasks at hand — planning, redecorating, preparing for the birth of your child with joy and excitement. But they're not diversions at all. They are part of the important work of preparing for motherhood.

LINDSEY CAME TO my office three weeks after she found out she was pregnant. She was convinced that she'd made a huge mistake and had no business being a parent. She was seriously considering terminating the pregnancy, but her obstetrician wisely sent her to speak with me first. There was nothing physically wrong with her that would prevent her from having a healthy baby. She and her husband were financially secure and had a close relationship. As much as anyone can be, she was in a good place to have a baby. So what was the problem?

"I can't have a baby. I'll be a terrible parent," she said, sitting on the edge of her seat and gripping the arms of the chair.

I looked inquisitively at her. "What makes you say that?"

"I just realized that my own childhood was so painful that I have no idea what being a good parent looks like. I'm so afraid

I'm going to be just like my own parents even if I don't want to be. I think the best thing for me to do is never to have kids."

Lindsey grew up in a family with an alcoholic father. When he drank, which was often, he became both verbally and physically abusive to Lindsey's mother and the kids. When Lindsey called home to tell her parents the good news, she got into a screaming match with her father. She felt disappointed, angry, and scared. She was convinced that the family legacy would haunt her forever.

Having negative thoughts, even if they make you sad, is not necessarily bad — and they don't make you a bad person. Negative experiences in childhood, though painful, can help you choose a different path in your current life. Lindsey and I spoke about what it would be like to have a baby and about her fears that the stress of listening to her baby crying, changing countless dirty diapers, and getting up for two o'clock feedings would make her act the way her parents had. I assured her that although she had learned the wrong way to interact with children while she was growing up, it was possible to learn the right way now. I would help her walk through child rearing if she needed support and advice. She was not doomed to repeat the past.

Many women — and men — who come from troubled families worry that their childhood experiences will keep them from being the kind of parents they want to be. The idea that child abuse is inevitably passed through the generations isn't accurate. There are many ways in which new parents can help themselves not repeat the sins of their fathers and mothers. Realizing that you are at risk for repeating abuse is the first step toward getting the help you need. Speaking with a member of the clergy or a therapist, adopting your own individual spiritual practices, or reading some of the books available on childhood development and parenting can help you start to heal. Becoming a parent yourself may even give you the chance to reexperience your own childhood in a more joyful and kind way.

✂

I SAW AMY a couple of weeks after our lunch. She was feeling better, partly because of what had happened the night before. She'd had a dream in which Paige had appeared, holding an infant. Paige didn't talk or even move much, but the incline of her head and shoulder as she lovingly cradled the infant was all Amy needed. She realized that having a good mother is good training for motherhood, even if the teacher is no longer here. Amy carries her mother with her wherever she goes.

"I couldn't have been the success I am today if it weren't for Mom," she said, "even though she was gone right after I graduated from college." I remained quiet, and she continued. "And she was very right about the men in my life, even though I didn't much appreciate her comments." We both smiled at the memory of Paige's jokes about the men in her own life. "Her view of men is my view of men," she added. "And that guided me straight to Michael, thank heavens." I nodded.

"So I guess," she said, looking out the window, "she'll also guide me in ways I don't even know when the baby is born."

"She will," I said. "Your mom left you so much love and wisdom. I see her in your eyes, and I see her in how you live your life."

The baby has since arrived. She's adorable, of course, with her grandmother's dark brown eyes and her name, Paige.

✂

ALL OF US grow up determined not to do some of the things our parents did when we were young. I swore that when I had a daughter, I would never humiliate her on the occasion of her first bra. I may have the story wrong, but in my memory my mother stood me in the middle of the bra department of our local department store and announced at the top of her lungs, "My daughter needs help buying her first bra. Are there any that will fit someone who has very small breasts?" I wanted to open up a hole in the floor and disappear. Becoming a mother allows us the opportunity to get it "more right." One of the blessings of the generations is that we can hope to do a better job than our parents did, just as they tried to do a better job than theirs. I, of course, managed to get it right with my daughter. She simply refused to go to the store with me and took a girlfriend instead.

Too Much of a Good Thing

Maggie was a woman used to being in control and at the top. But now, in my office for the first time, she looked scared and uncertain. An executive in a Fortune 500 company, Maggie was beautiful, smart, successful, and single. At the age of thirty-eight, she decided that since she had not found the right guy but wanted to have a child, she would pursue motherhood on her own. It wasn't easy for Maggie to get pregnant. She endured two long years of tests and shots, artificial insemination, and more tests and treatments. For the first time in her life, she was up against her biology. As a college soccer player, she'd felt in control of her body, and since then it had always done what she'd asked of it. This "failure" felt to Maggie like some kind of judgment for mistakes she had made during her youth and for being so single-minded about her career.

Finally, with the help of an excellent fertility group in town, Maggie found herself pregnant. She was first relieved and then ecstatic. The trouble began when, at about twelve weeks, Maggie learned that she was having twins. This threw her for a loop. She had already planned everything in her mind: the baby's room, the nanny, and the (only slightly) modified work schedule. She was not prepared for doubling the number of babies.

Until she got the news about the twins, Maggie had seen herself as a heroine, bravely marching by herself into motherhood, shoulders back and head held high. Now she was paralyzed with anxiety and saw herself as a selfish person.

"I really was ready to have a child," she told me. "I worked hard to make my dream come true." So why did she feel so bad? "When I tell people I'm having twins, they are so excited for me. They tell me stories of their friends and how much fun it is. They pass on helpful tips about living with chaos." Maggie gave me a look. "I can barely paste a smile on my face during these conversations. They are thinking about the adorable twosome, and I am thinking about the fact that my life is about to be over."

Maggie needed some help in coping with her changed reality. Of course, she is not a bad person, but she was right about how hard it is to have twins. The fact that everybody around her was bubbling with enthusiasm made her feel a lot worse than she should have, because she viewed her anxieties and worries as a sign of bad character. Let's call Maggie's situation a double whammy. Maggie is a perfectionist, accustomed to success at every step. But she hadn't found a life partner and had made the decision to plunge into motherhood alone. Then she couldn't get pregnant easily and had to undergo years of painful and emotionally exhausting treatment. When she finally did conceive and was appropriately happy, she got the news of the twins. That wasn't in the plan, and she could not adjust immediately.

In addition, she couldn't twist her feelings to conform to the response of friends and family, who were putting a good face on what was a difficult reality. Multiple births are becoming much more common because of the widespread use of fertility treatments, but they are a burden. In addition, Maggie would be carrying this burden alone, without the support of a partner. Maggie wasn't crazy. She is a smart and effective woman who was venturing into a new world, and she wasn't feeling brave. It is hard for a woman to give up her autonomy and self-reliance when she becomes pregnant. Luckily, nine months gives her time to adjust to the new reality. But there is not enough time in the world for a successful, demanding perfectionist to adjust to the idea of two babies at once. When Maggie came to see me, she needed reassurance that her panic about the future was not unrealistic. She also needed a reality check about her feelings. I told her that her concerns were legitimate and that a woman can want to be a mother but not want to be a mother of twins. Most of all, Maggie needed help in devising coping strategies for the future.

Her fantasies of motherhood were based in part on the fact that her mother had been aloof with her. Her mother hadn't given her much attention or much snuggling. Maggie dreamed of passing long, quiet days in the house with a sweet baby. That fantasy may have mothers of small children chuckling, but the fact is that there are a lot of quiet, snuggly moments with a first baby. Those moments are harder to find when there are older kids in the house and almost impossible when there are two infants.

The moral of Maggie's story is that being scared or intimidated by future motherhood does not mean that a woman is nuts — she may just be a little more realistic than most of us. A reality check that validates all feelings — positive and negative — is just what the expectant mother needs.

☙

THERE IS NO "right" way to feel when you are expecting a baby. No one else will have the same pregnancy experience as you. There will be good times and not-so-good times. Accepting your feelings will help you to have a less stressful nine months. It is also important to have a strong support system — people who will let you talk about your ambivalence, your fears, and your joys without passing judgment. Having a baby is a major transition in life — one that requires patience, understanding, and openness to new experiences.

2

The First Trimester

Extraordinary things happen to your body during pregnancy. Until you've been pregnant, you can't know how easy or how hard it will be for you. And every pregnancy is different, even for the same woman. Some women love every minute of being pregnant. Their skin glows, they have boundless energy, and they feel more beautiful and sexual than ever before. These lucky women say that they have never felt better in their lives. For others pregnancy is a struggle. The morning sickness that occurs morning, noon, and night seems as if it will never end. There are backaches, stretch marks, and varicose veins. For those women, those nine months seem to last longer than any other nine months in their lifetime.

Along with the physical challenges that come with pregnancy, there are also emotional ones. The transition from prepregnancy to motherhood requires psychological adaptation. Realizing that conflicts and strong new feelings are normal can help make the changes easier to accept and to work through.

During the first trimester in particular, the physical demands of pregnancy can be psychologically overwhelming.

Over time, I have found that women face three types of challenges as their bodies begin to adapt to the demands of growing a baby: the physical ones brought about by the enormous hormonal swings of pregnancy; the psychological challenges of changing relationships within the family and with the world; and the loss of identity many women experience when they realize that they are no longer in control of their bodies or their minds. This chapter addresses these challenges.

The Conspiracy of Silence

Recently, I received a phone call from my friend Janice, who was pregnant. Janice had suffered two miscarriages in the first trimester, and all of her friends were concerned about her ability to carry this baby to term. When I called her back, the first thing I asked was, "Are you okay?"

"I'm terrible," she said. I held my breath. Her voice made me think she had lost the baby. When she complained about her bad morning sickness, I was relieved.

An award-winning journalist, Janice had put off getting pregnant until she finished a major investigative series for a local newspaper. At first she couldn't conceive, and then she miscarried. This time Janice seemed to be holding on to the pregnancy. But she was also struggling with the hormonal symptoms common in early pregnancy. She couldn't think straight, she was so tired she couldn't get out of bed when her alarm went off, and she had terrible morning sickness. Her emotions were changing from moment to moment, and she had come to the conclusion that her career was over.

I did my best to comfort her. I told her that the hormones

that protect the fetus also can produce many of the symptoms she was experiencing. She understood that intellectually, but my generalizations didn't touch her where she lived. She told me that friends who didn't have children couldn't empathize with her; they couldn't imagine it being that bad. They thought that she shouldn't complain. After all, this pregnancy was working, unlike her earlier attempts, and they'd been present for her tearful losses so many times. She imagined that they were thinking, "You shouldn't be complaining. You tried so hard to have this baby. You should be grateful. I can't believe you're being so selfish." She felt extraordinarily guilty for wanting a baby so badly and now being so miserable.

Nobody had said to her, "Janice, you're not a bad person; it's not your fault. Yes, you feel miserable. Sometimes I felt miserable, too. But you *will* feel better."

Then she told me that her writer friends had warned her that she would never again write the way she had before getting pregnant. Her mind would be permanently changed by motherhood; she'd have "mommy brain," and she'd better prepare for life without the great career she had begun. Even if she *was* able to think intelligently again, she would be so consumed by diapers, baby food, and Barney that there wouldn't be time to express what she thought.

"What?" I yelled into the phone.

"Well," she said, "isn't that true?"

By now I was angry. I reminded her of the prize-winning writers who had children, the full-time volunteers who had children, the women heads of state who had children. Janice was in a weakened condition, and she was vulnerable to old wives' tales. We talked for about an hour, and then she asked me why nobody else had talked to her the way I did.

Why do so many mothers keep the whole story of pregnancy

from their daughters? Why do so few women help each other by admitting their fears, worries, and ambivalence during pregnancy? Why isn't there a body of honest lore and comfort for women embarking on motherhood to draw on? There's certainly a difference between telling the truth and scaring a new mother. There's no need to overdramatize how difficult life is when you have children. But there's also no need to pretend that it's easier than it really is. That approach only sets women up to feel like failures when things don't go as smoothly as they appear to for everyone else. In response, women struggle to keep their mouths shut, not wanting to admit that they are the only ones who don't have a clue about this pregnancy and parenthood thing.

I think this conspiracy of silence has many causes. The first is amnesia — biology's way of keeping the species going. If every mother remembered in detail all the woes and pains of pregnancy and delivery, *Homo sapiens* would have died out long ago. But amnesia isn't enough to explain the silence. Perhaps people don't want to scare pregnant women or make them hyperalert to all the possible downsides of pregnancy and motherhood. Or maybe they don't want to admit that being a mother is a very hard job.

One of the biggest reasons for the silence, I think, is that there is a cultural taboo against mothers having mixed feelings. Pregnant women are icons in our society: strangers touch their bellies, people on elevators give them advice on breastfeeding and diapers, and their every public action is scrutinized. Icons don't throw up all day or feel overwhelmed about the future. Mothers are sacred; they will always love us, and they will always think we're wonderful. If we allowed mothers to be real people with real feelings — if we admitted that mothers sometimes don't enjoy being pregnant or don't feel like taking care of their children — we'd also have to admit that sometimes our own mothers might not have been all that happy with us, every minute of the day.

I was reading *People* magazine recently and saw many beautiful movie stars beaming at the camera, showing off their big bellies or looking just wonderful as they held their newborns. It made me feel bad for all the pregnant women and new mothers who had the time to leaf through this magazine. I wanted to call out to them and say, "Don't imagine that's what you're supposed to strive for. They are ten deep in help! The makeup and hair people spent hours on them! They are crying just like you, and their episiotomies hurt them, too. They just aren't telling. And the reason they're back in their tiny jeans six weeks after delivery is that their personal trainers went to the hospital with them."

I discussed all this with Janice, who admitted the secret name she and her husband had given the fetus: TDC (That Damned Critter). I let out a whoop of laughter, and I could hear in her voice such a sense of relief that she had told me everything and I still wanted to be her friend. She was beginning to realize that her feelings were part and parcel of being pregnant, and she felt a lot better about her future — as a writer and as a mother.

Loss of Separateness

Once you become pregnant, you are no longer a single, autonomous person. Some other being inhabits your body, and from the beginning of pregnancy, "it" exerts subtle and not-so-subtle influences. Your hormones begin to change your body even before you're aware you are pregnant. Some women actually feel the embryo implant in the uterus about ten days after conception. When this happens, you realize that you are no longer alone in your body.

You may truly enjoy carrying your baby. For some women, nothing compares to the feeling of a baby moving inside them. This movement can be comforting, reminding you that your baby is a living being waiting to be born.

Yet from the first moment of pregnancy, every decision you make may have an influence on the embryo, fetus, and infant. Because of the potential risk of harm, you may no longer drink alcohol, take the medications you want, or eat raw fish or lunchmeat. Even tuna fish is suspect, due to the potential of mercury poisoning. You used to be able to stay out and watch the ten o'clock movie until it was over, but now you find that you fall asleep before the ten o'clock movie even starts. If you are nauseated, foods that used to be pleasurable are unbearable even to think about.

Even if you have tried hard to get pregnant, it can be difficult to accept how your body has been taken over and is focused on growing a baby in the most efficient way. If you do not eat well-balanced, nutritious meals or take vitamins to supplement your diet, the baby will use the nutrients your own body needs. The baby's needs always come first.

Sometimes all you can think about is getting the baby out of your body. You would give anything to be able to sleep on your stomach, eat pizza without heartburn, or get through a whole night without waking up. Especially during the second half of pregnancy, the thought of having your body back occupies your mind almost as much as longing to see what your baby will look like.

Particularly during the first trimester — the name given to approximately the first three months of pregnancy — early hormonal events are driving both the physical and the emotional changes. You may not even know you are pregnant, but your body is already adapting. I remember the first time I became pregnant, I was aware of being unusually thirsty before I even saw the stick change color. I had no clue as to why I was having that strange symptom. When that feeling returned with subsequent pregnancies, I knew immediately what was going on and went straight for a pregnancy test. Some women report losing their taste for coffee all of a sudden or feeling terribly fatigued. These and other "unusual" symptoms may occur within days of conception. Just imagine how powerful those early hormonal changes are. It's not surprising that they cause our bodies and our minds to be affected in profound ways.

Hormones and Their Effects on Your Moods

Before you know that you're pregnant, and long before anybody else knows, your body knows. Not only do we have the largest brain of any animal, but we also have a number of other highly organized systems — notably our immune and endocrine systems — that mobilize and perform critical functions. Unlike the brain, these systems can't help us pass an algebra test or do well on our SAT, but without them, we wouldn't even be around.

Think for a moment about the immune system — the cells and organs in your body that battle germs. It works like the most amazing defense department you could imagine. The instant a virus or bacterium attacks, your immune system is mobilized. Viruses and bacteria can survive only if they multiply, which is what they do immediately upon arriving in your body. Because viruses change shape and chemistry quickly, your body does not have cells to fight every virus on the planet. Instead, you have smart cells that learn very quickly the shape and chemical makeup of the invaders. These cells morph into other cells that stop the invaders from multiplying. You begin to feel better, and in time you're back to normal.

The endocrine system is equally elaborate; it performs numerous critical life functions but also has the ability to become uniquely focused the moment you are pregnant. Over the next nine months, the makeup of the hormones that enter your bloodstream changes, depending on the stage of pregnancy and what your body needs to grow and protect the developing baby. These hormones are engaged at the moment of conception; their job is to promote the safety and growth of your baby. Regardless of how they make you feel, they will be protecting your baby for the next nine months.

In early pregnancy, progesterone is secreted by the cells in the ruptured follicle of the ovary, the first source of this vital hormone. HCG (human chorionic gonadotropin), produced by the placenta, is the primary hormone responsible for promoting this ovarian production of progesterone. HCG is the hormone that maintains the pregnancy in its earliest stages, and it is this hormone that home pregnancy tests measure. The level of HCG peaks at around two months.

Once the fertilized egg has implanted in the uterus, the developing placenta takes over the secretion of the hormone progesterone. The placenta is also responsible for the secretion of estrogen, another hormone important to the health of the pregnancy. The levels of estrogen and progesterone in your blood continue to rise exponentially until delivery and have profound effects on your body and emotions. With the delivery of the placenta after the birth of the baby, these hormones drop precipitously, akin to driving a car off a cliff.

The problem is that the hormones that flood your bloodstream may make you feel awful. In early pregnancy in particular, HCG may be responsible for the terrible morning (sometimes all-day) sickness that some women experience and for their overwhelming fatigue. Estrogen and progesterone may account for the moodiness and tearfulness that are particularly noticeable in the early and late stages of pregnancy.

As a newly pregnant woman, you're told that these symptoms will pass. Common wisdom states that after the first trimester, the nausea and tiredness will go away. When I tell women that myself, however, I don't see smiles of relief. It's cold comfort to be told that something is transitory when you're suffering right now. It's almost impossible to imagine that you will ever feel better when you feel so lousy. And for a few women, the physical discomfort of early pregnancy lasts much longer than twelve weeks. Fortunately, this is not true for most women, who may experience some relatively mild discomfort (although it may not seem mild at the time) that is easily forgotten once they're through the worst of it. It's a good thing human beings have short memories, or many women would never have more than one child.

One of the issues women in the first trimester face is that, even though they may be over the moon about having a baby, and even though they know that this will be the best-loved child on the planet, they don't feel good. And you can't control how you feel. So when a relative or a good friend calls to share in your delight, it's hard to have a long, happy conversation if you've just finished throwing up. It's also hard to fix or even eat dinner, even though you never missed a meal before.

There are also cognitive changes that take place as a result of your geared-up hormones. Many women complain of forgetfulness or a foggy feeling. In some studies of menopausal women, the hormone progesterone, which is predominant in early pregnancy, has been shown to have negative effects on memory when given alone or in combination with estrogen, although other studies have shown no effect. Whether progesterone has an effect or not, all of your hormones, changing so rapidly, affect your body and the way you think and feel. This can result in your not being able to remember where you put your keys five minutes ago — which can be frustrating if you're on your way to a prenatal appointment. Whereas once you may have just blown it off and retrieved your extra set of keys from the kitchen drawer, now it feels as if the world is ending, and you find yourself standing in the middle of the kitchen sobbing.

After delivery, many women complain of "mommy brain" while they're breastfeeding. This is described as feeling totally stupid and unable to remember things you could previously recall in a snap. A scientist I treated wondered whether she'd ever be able to work in the lab again. Once she'd known how to sequence DNA, and now she was having trouble remembering her cat's name. Memory loss may be associated with low levels of estrogen during breastfeeding. Some research suggests that estrogen may be useful in maintaining cognitive functioning. For instance, estrogen has been studied as a treatment for memory decline in postmenopausal women.

It's no wonder, with all of the hormonal changes occurring in your body over a relatively short period of time, that your brain is affected. This hormonal bath, which is so beneficial to the baby, is sometimes very hard for you to take. The tiredness, the moodiness, and the nausea often overshadow the expected excitement of finding out you're going to have a baby. And when you don't feel the joy you imagined, you may think that there's something wrong with you and that you're not going to be the wonderful mother you thought you'd be. Everyone else feels ecstatic when they're pregnant. Why is it so hard for you to focus on the thought of holding your sweet baby in your arms? This is the reality that many women live with for the first twelve weeks.

Loss of Control

Cynthia had a life many women would envy. She had accomplished her career goals, had received every promotion she'd ever tried for, and felt as if there was nothing she couldn't do if she put her mind to it. Now in her mid-thirties and married to a man she adored, she was ready for kids. Like many things in her life, getting pregnant came easily to her. After only a couple of months of trying, she and her husband learned the good news: they were going to have a baby. Cynthia assumed that she'd be as successful at being pregnant as she had been in the rest of her well-accomplished life. And then all hell broke loose.

Cynthia called her mom for help. "I can't stop crying," she told her mother. "I know I'm supposed to be happy, and I think I am, but I'm not. This pregnancy thing was a really bad idea. I throw up all the time, I can't work, and I feel like a total fat slob. I'm nowhere big enough for maternity clothes, but I can't button my pants. All I'm comfortable in are sweatpants. Can you see me wearing those to work? I can't get more than ten feet from the bathroom because I feel like I'm going to vomit all the time. People are starting to get annoyed that I'm not available at my job. Everybody gets pregnant and seems fine. Why can't I do this? I'm so afraid that I'm going to be a lousy mom." This litany of misery was spoken between sobs and gulps of air.

"Oh, I'm sure you'll be a great mom," Cynthia's mother said. "We're all so excited to have our first grandchild. You'll be fine. The early part can be a little rough, but everybody gets through it." Cynthia's mom had always been a huge supporter of her eldest daughter. She'd seen Cynthia succeed at everything she'd tried. It was hard for her to understand that now Cynthia was having a really hard time.

"You know, I felt a little emotional and had some morning sickness when I was pregnant with you," she said. "But mostly it's just so exciting to know that there's a life growing inside of you. I couldn't wait to hold you and to sing to you. The day your baby is born will be one of the happiest days of your life."

Cynthia replied, "But, Mom, I don't just have morning sickness; I'm sick all the time. I open the refrigerator door and start gagging. It's all I can do to keep water down. I can't even brush my teeth. Putting a toothbrush in my mouth makes me vomit. I don't think I can do this. I'm only eight weeks' pregnant, and if it stays this bad much longer . . ." Another wail erupted on the other end of the line.

"Sweetie, having some nausea is normal this early in the pregnancy. It will get better, I promise. Try eating some saltines before you get out of bed — that always helped me."

Cynthia had to cut the call short as she ran to the toilet with dry heaves.

Cynthia's morning sickness was just the beginning of her anxiety. She was feeling totally out of control. Her body felt like an enemy, and her worries about the health of the fetus began to consume her. She started surfing the Web for information on fetal abnormalities in older mothers. She began to think that her bouts of throwing up could hurt the baby, and she started having nightmares about what else could go wrong. Her dreams were filled with images of babies that looked like squirrels. Sometimes she dreamed that she had given birth to an alien.

Cynthia had one of the earliest possible fetal tests for detecting genetic abnormalities. She went to a specialist for chorionic villus sampling (CVS) at week eleven of the pregnancy and paid several hundred dollars out of her own pocket to get preliminary results within forty-eight hours. Although those results appeared to be normal, she was only calmed for a day. The technician told her to remember that even though the early results were good, something could still show up as abnormal down the line. She spent the next two weeks anxiously awaiting the final test results, which showed that everything was indeed fine. Cynthia felt better — for about a week. Then she began to imagine all the things that she possibly could have done to harm her baby, even though it seemed to be genetically fine. Was the bath water too hot? Had she eaten too much tuna before she'd gotten pregnant? Was she at risk for having a stillborn child?

Cynthia called her doctor repeatedly, asking for more tests. That's when her doctor suggested that she get in touch with me. She came to me in a panic; her fears about the well-being of her baby were overwhelming. She had been used to knowing exactly how she was going to function on any given day. Now, all of a sudden, she couldn't predict even whether she'd be able to get out of bed in the morning. Would she be able to sit through her eleven o'clock meeting, or would she have to get up several times to vomit? How could she bear not knowing for certain that everything would work out perfectly with her baby? Having a healthy baby wasn't something she could accomplish just by doing everything "right." She would have to learn to accept that having a baby carried some medical risks, but also that those risks were small. And although she could do some things to increase her chances of having a healthy baby, worrying wasn't going to help her at all.

Over the course of a couple of sessions, we were able to deal with Cynthia's fears and with her sense of loss: the loss of being able to guarantee the outcome of her pregnancy, and the loss of her perception that she had total control over her life. Cynthia was having an especially hard time adjusting to the fact that she was no longer in charge of herself, her moods, her anxieties, and her brain. Often for a high achiever like Cynthia, good is not good enough; perfection is the only option. An important life-long lesson for anyone about to become a parent, however, is that good is often the best you can do, and many things about having and raising children are simply out of our control. To try to control things that are ultimately uncontrollable can only leave you feeling anxious and frustrated.

Pregnant While Parenting

Even women who have gone through a first pregnancy and who thought they'd learned these lessons can be caught short the next time around. Every pregnancy is different, even for the same woman. If your first pregnancy was hard, it can be helpful to know that the next one might be easy. But for some women, just the opposite is true. For Caroline, the second time around came as a big disappointment.

❧

CAROLINE WAS TWENTY-FOUR when she became pregnant with her first child. She was thrilled; she had always wanted to be a mother, and she hoped she'd be fortunate enough to have three or four children. The first pregnancy was, in her words, "a piece of cake. I never felt better. I loved being pregnant. My mood was actually better when I was pregnant — none of that moody PMS stuff to deal with. And I loved being able to eat without worrying about getting fat. I think I looked great pregnant, and my husband thinks so, too." With a big grin she confessed, "I don't know if everyone feels this way, but the sex was great. My husband loved it that my breasts got bigger, and there must be something about all the extra blood flow or something, because I felt really sexy the whole time."

Caroline was fortunate that her delivery was as easy as her pregnancy. But her second pregnancy was a different story. Being pregnant with a two-year-old at home made it hard for her to take care of herself as she had during her first pregnancy. Two-year-old Ryan didn't understand that Mommy was tired and wanted to take a nap instead of telling him stories, making him a peanut butter sandwich, or helping him finger-paint. And even though Caroline became nauseated at the sight of food, she still needed to prepare dinner for the family.

Caroline was part of a playgroup with other mothers of young children. One of the mothers, Toya, was in her thirties. Toya recognized the exhaustion in Caroline's face and asked if there was anything she could do to help.

"You look really, really tired," Toya said. "I heard you just found out you are expecting your second child. It's hard, isn't it, to manage with a toddler in tow?"

"You're so right," Caroline replied. "I'm only about six weeks' pregnant, but I don't know how I'm going to make it. All I want to do is sleep. But Ryan has decided he needs to wake up at six in the morning, and he also is trying to give up his afternoon nap. That nap is the only thing that saves me at the moment."

Caroline looked as if she was about to cry. At the same instant, Ryan started screaming as another little boy decided it was time to hit him over the head with a dump truck. Smiling through her tears, Caroline said, "I'm going to lose it. I don't know whether to laugh or cry. It's like this on a daily basis. I so enjoyed my first pregnancy; I thought I'd have three or four. There's just no way I could do this again."

Toya volunteered, "Let me go sort out the screaming for you, then we'll sit down and have a talk. It's really different when there's more than one at home to deal with, but not impossible. I've got some secrets I can share with you."

Being pregnant when you have other children at home is very different from being pregnant for the first time. What may seem like anxiety, depression, or illness may in reality be a reaction to the physical demands of pregnancy and the stress of caring for small children. Sleeping late on the weekends is not an option when you've got kids who wake up at six in the morning. You still have to make pancakes and hot dogs, when even the smell of fresh laundry can send you running to the toilet. And being sleep deprived and nauseous while trying to follow your usual routine can make you feel incredibly irritable, overwhelmed, and despondent. You may feel as if having another child was the worst mistake you and your partner ever made.

❧

WOMEN ARE WAITING longer to have children, and they have more years of school and work behind them than ever before. They are accustomed to doing what they want, when they want. Early pregnancy is the opposite of control. In fact, you have no control over how your body responds to the hormonal changes and the new life growing inside you. Your sister will tell you that she felt great, and your next-door neighbor will swear that she's never been sicker in her life. You can read all the books you want, but until *you* are pregnant, there's no way to know what pregnancy will be like for you. Even if it's your second or third or even fourth pregnancy, you're never quite sure how it will go. It's possible that each pregnancy will be slightly or even very different.

So give yourself a break and know that 99.9 percent of the women who have ever had children have experienced many of the same things you are feeling. That won't make the symptoms go away, but it might make you feel better about yourself and your ability to cope.

❦

I WAS SPEAKING with a pregnant friend not long ago. We agreed that, long before beginning Lamaze classes, women need what we wanted to call "truth in pregnancy sessions" to provide honest, down-to-earth coping advice. "We'll call them TIPS," my friend said. This idea inspired me to include a TIPS section at the end of many of the chapters in this book. Some of these ideas will be reminders of coping strategies for the difficulties that many women encounter at every stage of pregnancy and during the postpartum period. Some will be plain old tips. They'll all be honest, because honesty calms worries, reduces anxiety, and helps alleviate the sense of aloneness that troubles so many new mothers.

· TIPS ·

1. *To tell or not to tell.* Many couples choose not to tell friends and family that they are pregnant until after the first trimester. Their thinking is that if something goes wrong early on, it will be easier not to have to let everyone know that the pregnancy didn't work out. They may worry about the awkward questions and the awkward answers. Some couples are so overcome with excitement that they tell everyone who will listen. They have been waiting for this day and can't wait to let the whole world know.

There is no right or wrong way to handle this. Maybe a course somewhere in the middle is best. It's difficult to keep your pregnancy a complete secret, especially when you start turning down wine with dinner or have to skip meals because of nausea. More important, if you have a miscarriage or some other problem with the pregnancy, you will need the support and comfort of those who love you.

I have counseled many couples who suffered the pain of a miscarriage alone because they had not told friends or family about the pregnancy. Losing a pregnancy is a lonely road, even with the help of those close to you. So I suggest telling close family and your closest friends. They can be in on the joyful secret and will enjoy hearing all the details of the early ultrasounds and hearing the baby's heartbeat. This will make them feel special, and if the worst happens, they will be there to share in your sorrow and pain. They will understand what you have lost because they were there for the early joy.

2. *What to read, whom to believe.* When you join the pregnancy club, other women can't wait to tell you their stories: what they did, what books they read, what you absolutely can't do, and what you absolutely must do. People will tell you what you should eat and how much you should (or shouldn't) exercise; they will advise you on every inconsequential detail imaginable.

Even strangers feel that they have the right to judge a woman for what she does while she is pregnant. During my last pregnancy, I was at a restaurant with my husband. It was late in my third trimester, and I was feeling very big and very cranky. In Texas, the frozen margarita is the state alcoholic beverage, and there's nothing better than a big bowl of chips and *queso* (cheese) and a cold, salty margarita. I'd given margaritas up during my pregnancy except for an occasional sip. That night my husband and I agreed that I would order one and we'd split it. Both the baby and I might get a good night's sleep.

When the waiter asked what I'd like, I said, "A frozen margarita, please, with salt."

He replied, "I'm sorry, ma'am. I'm afraid I can't serve you that."

"Why not?" I asked, thinking that the margarita machine must be broken.

"Well, you're pregnant, and it's not good for your baby."

I was stunned. I was already in a bad mood, and it was quickly getting worse. "Excuse me? It's none of your business whether I have a drink or not."

"I'm not going to serve a pregnant woman," he said, then walked away.

I was seething. I was ready to let him have it, explaining that my husband and I are both physicians and know very well the risks of drinking during pregnancy. I would do nothing to harm our baby and probably would have had no more than a sip or two. As a matter of fact, alcohol used to be given intravenously to stop premature contractions. I stood up, about to call him back over to the table for a medical lesson. Being the calmer of the two of us, my husband guided me out of the restaurant.

When you are pregnant, everyone feels entitled to an opinion about what you should or should not do. If you try to listen to everyone and follow all the advice you read in books, you will lose your mind. The most important person on this journey is your doctor or midwife. Find one you trust and listen to him or her. Different doctors have different advice. Some say it's okay to have an occasional glass of wine; others say absolutely not. It's important that you feel comfortable with your doctor. If you feel more secure with a doctor who is strict about what you should and should not eat, she is the doctor for you. If you prefer a physician who is more relaxed and doesn't have rigid rules, that's your guy. If you don't feel good about your physician, find another one. Every doctor has been fired at one point or another, and we don't take it personally. And once you find a health care provider you like, just smile when your next-door neighbor tells you that her doctor told her exactly the opposite of what yours told you. Then thank her for her advice and change the subject. You have enough to think about without second-guessing every decision you and your doctor make.

3

The Second Trimester

The beginning of the second trimester of pregnancy typically puts to rest the physical discomforts of the first twelve weeks. Many women report that they are able to spend less time in the bathroom and more time enjoying the wonders of their changing bodies. The relief from morning sickness and other symptoms and the joy of family and friends enables most women to join in the celebration of the upcoming event. The focus shifts from how lousy they feel to happily anticipating the baby's first kick. It's hard to remember just how hard it was to wake up every morning nauseous or how worried they were that they'd never be able to do this for nine months.

As you become more accustomed to the hormonal changes, it's great not to feel at war with your body. Estrogen and progesterone levels are rising slowly, and HCG is no longer playing a major role. Energy returns along with the ability to think clearly for more than a nanosecond. Sleep is better as your uterus starts to grow up out of your pelvis and there is less pressure on your bladder (for the moment). You may finally start to look pregnant and can stop worrying that people think you've just gotten fat. Worries about miscarriage lessen, and there is the excitement of telling everyone you're about to become a mother.

At this time, women often start to think concretely about the future and to plan for all the changes that will take place in just six months. That isn't long in a person's life, but these particular six months are packed with wishes, dreams, and worries. As reality sets in, your relationship with your partner will take on a new intensity. Where there was once only the two of you, there will soon be three, or even four. Even in the best of marriages, adding another person to the family changes the way the partners interact with each other. Both begin to think about the responsibilities of parenthood. At this stage of the pregnancy, the ultrasound shows a perfectly formed human being, with fingers, toes, and kicking feet. Sometime during the second trimester, you will even be able to tell the sex of the baby if you want to know it.

At three months, you will probably feel safe telling everybody that you are pregnant — as if you could hide it much longer. And in the following weeks, you can sense the baby moving inside you. I don't think anybody who has not been pregnant can imagine the experience of those first flutters. At first you're not sure whether you feel anything at all. Maybe it's gas or some strange "pregnancy feeling." And then it happens again, and this time you're sure that it's not your imagination.

But how to describe it? Like eyelashes blinking inside you or champagne bubbles tickling your belly? There really is no way to explain it, only to say it's exciting and awe-inspiring. Finally, it's so clearly a kick from a tiny foot or a punch from a tiny fist that you can't shrug it off any longer. You know that somebody is in there, and it's your child. Eventually, other people will be able to feel the baby kicking, but for the first few weeks, this is your private interaction with your baby, and it can't be shared with anyone else.

Feeling the baby move magnifies everything. The baby becomes a reality, and the pregnancy takes on new significance. You are now fully aware that a new person will be arriving, that you will be totally responsible for him or her, and that there's no going back. All of a sudden, the stakes of the decisions you make become much higher. You and your partner may have worked out the schedules and chores of a two-income couple, but what will happen when you have another person to worry about? Another person who's not going to contribute any income or help clean the house? A totally helpless, needy, demanding human being?

Not-So-Equal Partners

The reality is that men and women may respond differently to the approaching delivery. The mother-to-be may be totally focused on the baby and spend hours planning the nursery and looking at baby clothes. By contrast, the father-to-be may have trouble feeling emotionally connected to his wife's growing belly until he can feel the baby move. He just knows that she's changed in a way that he's not fully a part of. He may try to feel excited about the tiny socks his wife is holding up for him to admire, but he can't imagine how he'll ever be able to hold anything that small without breaking it. He's looking forward to throwing a football with his son; she's imagining singing lullabies.

Routines that at one time were second nature are now up for debate. A woman may shrug off her husband's habit of not calling when he's going to be late because she's perfectly happy calling for take-out when they're both home from work. But what will happen when she's at home and responsible for feeding a baby on a schedule? Will he start letting her know where he is and how to get hold of him? A husband may begin to worry about money when he considers the added expense of a baby or about life on one salary. Will his wife expect him to be able to make more money to pay all the bills? Will they need a bigger house? A nanny? What about medical bills? A kaleidoscope of thoughts and concerns crowds an expectant parent's mind.

Getting ready to have a child inevitably puts pressure on the relationship, and that is not a bad thing, because thousands of adjustments must be made on a daily basis when you have a child. Learning how to negotiate and compromise is crucial in any partnership, but never more so than when children are involved. The issues of parenting become more real in the second trimester. There will be conflicts and some disappointments. She may be imagining herself alone with her new family for the first few weeks; he may be expecting to return to work while his mother and mother-in-law hold down the fort. Both partners' expectations and concerns need to be shared and discussed.

❧

LIKE MANY YOUNG parents, Sally and Henry decided to keep their pregnancy quiet from as many people as possible until three months had passed. They told their immediate families but made them promise not to spread the news just yet. In the privacy of their home, Sally browsed the Internet, looking for the newest trends in maternity clothes, cribs, and baby wear. Now that she was over her mild nausea and fatigue and the news was out, Sally was all set to shop. Her list of things to buy for the nursery was prepared, she was ready to hit the maternity store at the local mall, and she had borrowed from her friends a foot-high pile of reading material, including a few baby-naming books.

Because Sally worked long hours in retail, she had a hard time finding time to go shopping with Henry, who had a nine-to-five job. But one evening they made a date to meet at the discount furniture outlet. Sally raced there from work, parked, and made a dash for the crib section. She checked out the inventory while she waited for Henry. Then she went to the rocking chair section. She figured Henry would find her there. No Henry. He was now half an hour late. Sally was momentarily concerned, then she walked over to check out the bassinets and got into a long and intricate conversation with a saleswoman about whether to get one with or without drawers. Finally, she was drawn into a conversation with a couple of other pregnant women about the relative virtues of the many strollers on display. All of a sudden, she realized that Henry was more than one hour late. Sally was truly worried. She called his cell phone and was relieved when he picked up. But she was not happy about where he was. Henry was having an after-work drink with his buddies. He had forgotten their date to pick out baby furniture.

When they met at home, Sally was hurt and crying; Henry couldn't believe he'd forgotten. He felt terrible about letting her down. After all, this baby had been their shared dream ever since they'd met in high school. Their child would be the first grandchild on Henry's side, and his parents were in a state of high excitement. Henry was absolutely wonderful when Sally didn't feel like cooking dinner — or eating it. He was a loving and attentive husband. Sally knew he'd be a great father. But this episode hurt her feelings and made her wonder if maybe he didn't really want a baby. Why wasn't he as excited as she was to get the nursery ready?

To make it up to her, Henry suggested that they snuggle on the couch and look up baby names. So there they were, sipping decaf iced tea and leafing through books. "Amanda?" she asked.

"Too trendy," he replied. "Kate," she said, thinking of a simpler name. "Hate it," he replied. This went on for nearly an hour, until Henry nixed Zoe, and Sally left the room in tears. Nobody finds the perfect name on the first try, but that night Sally slept with her back turned toward her husband.

She could not understand his attitude, and she began to feel more and more isolated from him, and angry. She had never doubted his love for her before, but Henry had changed, and for the first time they were not on the same wavelength. He felt distant and distracted, and she started to feel as if she were having this baby all by herself. Her life had changed tremendously; why hadn't his? The baby was all she could think of and talk about, but it didn't seem as if he was thinking about being a father at all. He acted as if life was just going to go on as usual.

Sally tried to hold back her tears when she told me this story. She had come to see me out of fear that her wonderful, close marriage was falling apart. This was not the man who'd cried when he'd seen the baby's heartbeat on the ultrasound screen. What kind of father was he going to be? Had they made a huge mistake? "What happened to my terrific husband?" she wondered.

❧

IT IS NOT an uncommon experience for women and men to process pregnancy in very different ways. Whereas women may feel excitement and dream about holding a sweet baby in their arms, men may feel anxiety about changing responsibilities, financial strain, and their wives' health. She may be willing to sacrifice her life for her child, but he may be worried about losing his wife and partner. As the baby becomes more of a reality for the pregnant woman during the second trimester, the father may still have a difficult time feeling connected to the child. He is committed to his wife and to their plans, but who is this person with whom his wife already seems to have a relationship? Men often are just as excited and concerned as women, but they may feel even less comfortable expressing negative feelings out of fear of not appearing supportive or strong.

I asked Sally to bring Henry in for a conversation. It was apparent to me that they were both good people and both invested in being parents, but they needed help expressing their positive and negative feelings to each other. Sally assumed that Henry felt exactly as she did, and when his behavior didn't match her feelings, she was confused. Henry was worried that talking to Sally about his difficulty getting excited about baby furniture would make her think he wasn't looking forward to being a father. They were both afraid that if they broached the subject of their conflict, their secure world would dissolve. Henry agreed to come to an appointment with Sally; he was looking forward to being able to talk about his mixed feelings and reestablishing a close connection with her before the baby arrived.

Henry had known that he wanted to be with Sally for the rest of his life the day he'd seen her across the table in chemistry lab. Even when they were dating, they would fantasize about having a large family, pick out names for their imaginary babies, and plan the number of girls and boys they'd like to have and in what order. But now, married for three years and expecting a real baby, Henry was feeling anxious. He worried about his ability to provide for his wife and baby. He liked his job all right, but he wasn't sure what kind of a future it offered. Henry and Sally had married right out of high school, and they both knew now that a better education would have improved their prospects. Henry wanted to be able to send his kids to college. Where was that money going to come from? He had grown up in a combative family, and his father had sometimes gotten violent. Henry remembered what it had been like to be scared of his dad. Would he be able to control his temper?

And what about his relationship with Sally? They had been a twosome for nearly a decade, devoting themselves completely to each other. A stranger was about to arrive — an interloper. Would he still get Sally's attention? Certainly, she didn't seem all that interested in him since she'd become pregnant, and she had no desire for sex. She seemed to be in her own world. "What's going to happen to us?" he thought. Henry was having a hard time adjusting to this new reality. That may have been why he "forgot" their shopping date and didn't like any of the baby names she suggested.

It's normal for both parents to be simultaneously thrilled and intimidated by the future. Raising children is a serious responsibility, and new parents have to grow up fast. Henry and Sally will probably do just fine. They are committed to each other, and even though Henry was not able to voice his concerns without some prodding, they communicate well. As they left my office, I wished them all the best. I told them that the most important thing they could do for themselves and the baby was to keep talking to each other, even when it was difficult. Children do best when their parents are able to work together to make tough decisions about the children's needs.

Sex and the Pregnant Parent

Marjorie found Miguel to be the single most adorable person on the planet, and Miguel returned the feeling. Every bit of Marjorie's body was attractive to Miguel and vice versa. The night they had met at a friend's party, it had been attraction at first sight, and they had spent more time in bed together than anywhere else. This powerful attraction had grown into a deep love over the following year, and they had been planning their wedding when Marjorie discovered she was pregnant. This didn't bother either of them; they were already thinking about a family and could afford a child right away. They began to plan for both a wedding and a baby.

Their sexual relationship, which had been their anchor, began to wane. Some nights, when Miguel approached her, Marjorie turned her back. She was exhausted from planning the wedding and the changes of early pregnancy. Miguel seemed to understand and, though disappointed by the decrease in their sexual activity, was willing to wait until Marjorie was feeling less exhausted. He'd heard from many of his friends that sex in early pregnancy is nearly nonexistent. He had thought they'd be different, since sex was so enjoyable for both of them, but Marjorie didn't have the energy for much of anything, especially physical intimacy.

The wedding took place sometime after Marjorie entered her second trimester. The morning sickness had disappeared, and Marjorie was feeling much better. So much better, in fact, that she was ready to resume their passionate relationship. Marjorie was starting to enjoy the changes in her body. She had a small swelling in her lower abdomen that wasn't too cumbersome, her breasts were full and seemed more sensitive to the touch, and it felt as if her whole body had more blood coursing through it. She liked the way she looked and felt sensual and ready to enjoy Miguel again.

But now Miguel wasn't feeling so sexy, and when he was, his body wouldn't cooperate. He found the changes in Marjorie's body frightening. It was obvious that she was pregnant, and the thought of putting his penis so near the baby during intercourse scared him. He was afraid that he would hurt the baby or his wife, and somehow having sex with a baby between them felt wrong. All of a sudden, Miguel was the one paralyzed and unable to perform. He started to avoid going to bed with Marjorie at night so that he wouldn't have to talk about his feelings.

So here they were, beginning their marriage, newlyweds who should be spending hours in bed, but with conflicting emotions concerning their desire for sex. And against all stereotypes, it was the woman who was craving physical intimacy and the man who was trying to avoid it. Marjorie recounted this story as she sat in my office in tears. She and Miguel loved each other, but what used to work for them so flawlessly — what was such an important connection for them — was now something they fought about constantly. They were trying to adjust to a new marriage and impending parenthood, and it felt like they would never enjoy sex again. To make matters worse, Marjorie had heard from her friends that after the baby was born, sex would become a distant memory. Marjorie worried that their marriage wouldn't last.

I asked her to return with Miguel, and the three of us spent several sessions talking about the realities of a new marriage and the challenges of continuing a sexual relationship during pregnancy. With some education and reassurance, they were able to resolve their conflicts, and their sex life returned, with all of its previous joy and passion. The third trimester posed some problems, as Marjorie started to feel more uncomfortable than sexy, but with some creative positioning, they were able to have sex up until she delivered.

❧

FOR MANY WOMEN, the first trimester is the time when the thought of sex seems least appealing. Fatigue and nausea are the biggest culprits in decreasing the frequency of sex. But for most couples, sex returns during the second trimester, and some women actually feel more sexual then than at any other time in their lives. Everything on a woman's body is swollen — her belly, her breasts, and her genitals — and this can make for some intense sexual pleasure. Her energy has returned, the nausea is gone, and, best of all, there is not yet a big belly to get in the way. Because the uterus is expanding, the uterine muscular contractions that are part of orgasm can be felt more intensely. This can be frightening for some women as the uterus becomes hard and contracted, sometimes for several minutes. Unless there is a risk for preterm labor, this is not in the least bit dangerous for the baby or the woman. (Your physician will tell you whether sexual intercourse is safe for you.)

It is not unusual for some men to feel squeamish about having sex with their pregnant wives. All of a sudden, the woman's body is not just for sexual pleasure but also for growing and nurturing a baby. It can be hard for the man to see the mother of his child as a sexual object. This mental block can be overcome with patience and talking about any fears and discomforts. For the woman, it is very important to remember that even though she is pregnant, she is still a sexual being. This awareness will be especially important when there is a real live baby interfering with the couple's romantic life. The best piece of advice? Don't talk about the baby in the middle of lovemaking. That will be a certain turnoff.

In some cases, a physician will tell a couple not to have sexual intercourse and advise the woman not to have an orgasm for fear of stimulating premature labor. If you receive this advice, there are many more ways to be intimate other than intercourse. Performing oral sex or bringing your partner to orgasm with your hand can be a way of being close and giving him pleasure. He may not be able to reciprocate, but back or foot rubs can feel awfully good when you're pregnant. And remember, pregnancy is a temporary condition; then the *real* challenges begin.

Losing Control of Your Shape

That new surge of energy in the second trimester is accompanied by important bodily changes, including a growing belly. Women often find their new shape a challenge to their body image, especially if they've been focused on exercise and maintaining a certain weight. For some women, the freedom to put on pounds is a relief; for others, the thought of gaining any weight at all can cause hours of anxiety. It seems impossible to expect a woman not to compare how much weight she has gained against some imaginary standard or not to compare herself to a friend who gained only twenty pounds and left the hospital in her blue jeans. There is a wealth of advice about how much weight you are supposed to gain, when, and by what means — and it is all very confusing.

When I think about weight gain during pregnancy, I'm reminded of the story "The Three Bears." I wish we could all agree on definitions of too little, too much, and just enough weight gain. But we're not bears in a storybook. What does "just enough" mean? Doctors offer instructions about weight gain, but even doctors differ in their advice. Books offer different numbers, and so do other women. We know that too much weight gain carries serious risks for gestational diabetes, hypertension, and a difficult delivery. And there certainly is the problem of losing the weight after you deliver. But there are also risks associated with too little weight gain, for both the mother and the baby. Whatever the magic number a pregnant woman is aiming for, one big complicating factor is appetite.

Pregnant women experience many extremes, and appetite is one of them. In the first three months, they don't want to look at food or think about it, except as something to stem the nausea. Then, along with all the other positive changes in the second trimester, comes what I think of as the Great Hunger. See a box of cookies and want one? The box is half-gone before you blink. Thinking about a scoop of ice cream? Oops, there goes the entire pint. All kinds of foods in the pantry mysteriously disappear, and partners are sent out on odd shopping sprees. I once ordered breakfast twice — the first serving of eggs, hash browns, and bacon just wasn't enough.

This never-ending desire for something to eat is difficult for women who are used to watching their weight. If controlling your appetite has been a way of life and suddenly that control is gone, you may get anxious: you're getting fat, and you can't help it. In a culture that awards a certain status to women who are thin and even superthin, putting on pounds can cause overwhelming distress.

Eating disorders, which are common among young women in our country, have to do with control and self-control. Being pregnant and having an eating disorder is a state of mixed signals: "I'm supposed to eat for the baby" and "I have to stop eating; I'm gaining weight." Reconciling these two competing signals presents an enormous challenge. It brings back all the issues that may have plagued you as a teenager and younger woman who struggled with eating issues. Body image, control, self-doubt, and perfectionism — these come into terrifying conflict with the body's need for ample nutrition, including carbohydrates and fats that have been banned from the most popular diets. It's impossible to tell a woman who has restricted her food intake all her life or has binged and purged that now, miraculously, she should allow herself to gain weight, which will make her feel horribly guilty — and fat.

❧

AMANDA'S OBSTETRICIAN CALLED me for a consult. She was worried about her patient, who was in her fifth month and had not gained enough weight. The doctor suspected that Amanda had had an eating disorder in the past, but she could not get the whole story from Amanda. She just had no appetite, Amanda said, as she tried to get out of her doctor's office. That no-appetite excuse had worked up through the beginning of the second trimester, but now the doctor was worried.

Amanda came to her appointment with me stylishly dressed in what appeared not to be maternity clothes. If I hadn't known she was pregnant, I wouldn't have looked twice at her belly. But now I was looking hard to find any evidence of a woman who was five months' pregnant. There was little more than a small bulge that I noticed when she sat down. Amanda was an extremely thin young woman; I could see why her obstetrician was worried.

I reviewed with Amanda the worries her doctor had relayed to me and her concern that Amanda might have an eating disorder. I told her how dangerous restricting her calories was for both her and the baby and that the baby would then use every available vitamin and mineral from Amanda's own body to continue growing. Amanda was en route to doing serious damage to her own body. She looked at me with chagrin and said, "I've tried to eat, but I just can't. The thought of gaining any weight is intolerable. I already feel so fat."

Given that I could barely tell she was pregnant, it was amazing to me that she would consider herself fat. But that is the nature of an eating disorder. The person has such an altered body image that when she looks in the mirror, she does not see what others see. Amanda truly saw a fat person when she looked in the mirror. It was impossible for her to eat enough to stay healthy.

Amanda is an extreme example of someone struggling with weight gain during pregnancy. But for any pregnant woman, weight gain can cause anxiety and discomfort. In our image-conscious society, any extra weight can be a cause of shame.

What is the answer? For women with severe eating disorders, psychotherapy and medication are mandatory. For women who gain large amounts of weight, putting themselves at risk, consultation with a nutritionist may be necessary. But for most women, the answer is to relax. Women rarely gain way too little or way too much weight. Your next-door neighbor may gain exactly twenty-three pounds and be praised by her physician for her excellent weight control. You gain thirty-five pounds and feel as if you've failed Pregnancy 101. But both of you will deliver healthy babies and will be able to get back to a normal weight with moderate diet and exercise.

How Can I Do This to Number One?

Cathy called for an appointment. She was having trouble sleeping, and she couldn't understand why. She had survived the first trimester at home with her two-year-old, and now she was feeling a lot better. But every time she began dozing off, she woke up with a start and couldn't get back to sleep. "I've been looking forward to this pregnancy," she told me when we met, "and it's going very well. The first time, I worried about every little thing, and it's such a relief to be able to enjoy being pregnant this time without so much anxiety getting in the way."

Cathy and her husband, Tony, had managed their finances

well enough for her to stop working when their first child, Samantha, was born. She loved being a stay-at-home mom. She had quit work a month before Samantha's due date and had had plenty of time to decorate the nursery and prepare for the new baby's arrival. Everybody had been happily surprised when Sam came a week early. Cathy had had a great pregnancy, and she and Samantha had been in harmony from the time the baby arrived. "I feel like I'm a great mom," she said.

Some children are just easy; they eat and sleep and gurgle and play, just like in the movies. Sam was one of them. I asked for a picture of Samantha, and there she was, dressed in an adorable sunsuit, with curly brown hair, big blue eyes, and a huge toothy grin. When Cathy pulled out the picture, she relaxed, and the anxiety she had carried into my office evaporated. Cathy gazed at this adorable child with such love that she almost fell into the snapshot.

When Cathy put the picture back into her wallet, I asked, "What do you think is bothering you? Things seem to be going so well." Cathy shrugged.

"How is Tony doing?" I asked. "Is he being supportive enough?"

Cathy gave me a big smile and said, "Absolutely! He's the best guy. When I was feeling really bad in the beginning of this pregnancy, he brought me crackers and took over Samantha the minute he got home from work. He is so excited about this baby — I can't tell you how much."

It was hard for Cathy to find the cause of her anxiety, so I asked her to tell me in detail about her day with Samantha. Cathy has organized her life around taking care of Sam and can't imagine anything better. Little Sam offers her mother bites of her favorite foods, and Cathy can get her to do anything she wants without a fight. No terrible twos here. Of course, Cathy felt bad that she wasn't up to doing everything she used to with Samantha, because she needed to nap a bit during the day, but even then they would cuddle together on the big bed.

Cathy had been looking forward to the return of energy with her second trimester so that she and Samantha could go back to their active schedule: classes in the morning, park in the afternoon, conversations in the car, creative play at home. Now they were constantly on the go again. Cathy loved being with her daughter and the closeness they shared.

"Is Samantha going to preschool when the baby arrives?" I asked, wondering whether it might be a good time for Sam to spend some time apart from her mother.

"I haven't decided," Cathy replied. "I know most people send their kids to preschool at two, but I'm teaching her a lot of things at home, and we go to all these classes for enrichment experiences. She doesn't seem too clingy, and I expose her to other kids at playgroup, so I'm not sure she needs it. Besides, I love her so much, I can't bear the thought of being away from her." With that, Cathy started to tear up.

It was then that we began to explore Cathy's feelings about abandoning her first child to take care of the new baby. As we talked, the tears flowed freely. "It's going to be so hard on Samantha when the baby arrives," she said. "I can't get away from the feeling that I am betraying her." Cathy looked up at me and said very quietly, "This is hard to admit, but I don't know how I'm ever going to love another baby as much as I do Sam."

As we talked, Cathy began to explore her fear that she would be leaving her darling little girl out in the cold and her worry that she'd be an inadequate mother to her second child. Cathy's relationship with her firstborn meant the world to her. She was the fourth of five children. Her mother had been loving and empathic, but exhausted. There had been so many demands on her that, as hard as she'd tried, she hadn't been able to spend much time individually with each of her children. When Cathy was a little girl, she had imagined herself as a mother someday. "I had this picture in my head of a mother bird trying to feed a nest full of baby birds, all with their beaks wide-open: five beaks up in the air, competing for food." That sounded like a pretty accurate account of what it feels like to be the fourth of five kids. "I always imagined being a mother with all the time in the world. I never wanted my kids to feel like they had to fight for my attention." Cathy knew that Samantha was about to get some competition, but her head also was filled with memories of the unmet needs she'd had as a child.

I tried to help Cathy see that Samantha, at age two, was no longer quite so fragile: she walked and ran, talked and played; she was starting to dress herself and knew what she wanted to eat. Perhaps she was ready for some time away from Mom. "You're right, it is hard for the first child to adjust to a new baby in the house," I said. "But it's an important part of growing up." Sam needed to begin the crucial process of separating from her mother so that she could become the self-assured and confident person she was meant to be.

The process of separation and individuation, the important step in obtaining growing independence from the mother, is a two-way street. It's a developmental task on both sides. Sure, the toddler will run back to Mommy for hugs and assurance that things are all right. But it's the mother's job to offer that comfort and then point the child gently in another direction. That can be painful to do. Having a child cuddle up in your lap, reach for your hand, and ask for help with a task are sweet times. But children need to grow up and away — that's how they become healthy, competent adults. Sometimes parents who are having a wonderful time with their little ones would love to stop the clock, but they can't do that.

Samantha was more than ready to begin this process. It is not developmentally healthy for a two-year-old to continue to believe that her every need will be met — that she will never have to wait for food if she's hungry or that everything she wants will automatically be handed to her. Learning to share her parents' time and energy with a new baby could help Sam to grow up. There may be some temper tantrums or regression to more babylike behavior — one last attempt to reclaim the most honored position — but ultimately things will calm down. To develop ethical relationships with others and to be otherwise successful in the world, a child must learn how to compromise, share, and wait her turn.

"You're a great mom, Cathy," I said. "You're going to be amazed at how much you are able to love this new child, and it won't diminish your love for Sam. What will be important for both of you is to make sure that you and Sam still have time alone with each other. And that doesn't mean with the baby in your arms. The two of you need to know that there will still be times when she has your undivided attention. That will go a long way toward helping her adjust to the new baby and to know she hasn't lost you. She will just have to learn how to share you."

I don't think Cathy left my office convinced of any of that, but at her next appointment she reported that she was beginning to sleep a bit better. Planning what her day would be like after the baby arrived was helpful. She was going to hire a sitter to care for the new baby part-time so that she and Sam could still go on outings they both enjoyed. And sometimes she would use the sitter for both children so that she could have some time to herself. I told her that I liked both ideas. It is critical that a new mother have time alone to pamper herself so that she will have enough energy to devote to her growing family.

· TIPS ·

1. *There are two parents.* Often the mother-to-be can become consumed with her pregnancy. It can be all she thinks about, worries about, and plans for. But it took two to get pregnant, and it will take two to raise the child. Remember that your partner may have his own fears and worries and that they may be entirely different from yours.

Any relationship needs communication and nurturing. Don't put your relationship on the back burner just because you're expecting. Now is the time to pay even closer attention to how you are doing as a couple. Being pregnant and having a baby will change your relationship in profound ways. It won't be just the two of you any longer, but in many ways you will need to form an even stronger team than ever before.

Set aside time each day to talk. Turn off the TV, put down the paper, and listen to each other. Asking how your partner is feeling and what he or she is thinking or worried about will keep you connected and working together. Don't assume that you know what your partner thinks or feels; many a good fight has started that way.

Men have special worries and concerns. Whereas Mom may be worried about her changing body and delivering the baby, Dad may be worried about financial matters or becoming second to the baby in his wife's affections. You are not just a pregnant woman, and your partner is not just a future dad. You are both still people who need love, attention, and intimacy. It may be hard to ignore your growing belly, but both of you need time to be more than just parents.

2. *Eating for two.* Weight gain during pregnancy can be traumatic for many women, but particularly for women who have an eating disorder. It is imperative that both you and your baby acquire adequate calories and nutrients during your pregnancy. Prenatal vitamins aren't enough to sustain either of you.

If the thought of gaining weight terrifies you to the point that it's affecting your food intake, ask your doctor to weigh you with your back to the scale. You don't need to know exactly what you weigh; just ask if you have gained sufficient weight since your last visit to ensure your baby's and your health.

To keep you feeling satisfied and decrease the feeling of being bloated or overfull, try eating many small, healthy meals throughout the day. Nibbling on healthy snacks can be a good way to get needed calories without feeling as if you're binging.

You may need to consult a nutritionist to help you plan your daily food intake. This way, you can be sure that you are getting the vitamins, nutrients, and calories that you need but not over- or undereating. You may be surprised at how much you need to eat to stay on a healthy weight-gaining track.

Purging is absolutely off-limits. Frequent vomiting can cause dehydration, loss of vitamins and minerals, and changes in electrolytes that are life threatening to you and your baby. There are medications that help control the urge to purge. Behavior therapy is also an excellent way to learn techniques to stop purging. Make sure you tell your doctor or midwife if this is a problem for you.

3. *Sex specifics.* Sex is possible during pregnancy and can be enjoyable despite what you may have heard. Don't let old wives' tales interfere with your intimate relationship. In some cases, your physician may tell you that sex is off-limits, but in most cases, you can have as much sex as you want. Sex toward the end of the pregnancy can actually stimulate labor.

During the first trimester, your sex drive may wane due to fatigue and nausea. But in the second trimester, as you begin to feel better, the increased blood flow throughout your body may make sex even more pleasurable. And unless you have some medical problem, it is in no way harmful to you or your baby.

Take advantage of your larger breasts by buying attractive lingerie to show them off. Your husband will be thrilled, and you may enjoy being bigger for a short while, too. (They do make sexy lingerie for pregnant women. You're not the only pregnant woman who's thinking about having sex.)

As your uterus becomes larger, penetration may become uncomfortable as the penis pushes up against your cervix. Changing positions may cause the penis to penetrate less deeply and prevent that problem. When your uterus grows too large, a face-to-face position may become impossible, but there are many other ways to have intercourse: rear entry, side by side, or with you sitting on top. This may be a time in your sex life when you can have fun trying new things.

Most important, keep your sense of humor. You both may feel awkward trying to maneuver around a large belly, but laughter can keep the tension to a minimum and make sex more enjoyable.

4

The Third Trimester

Highs and lows are all part of the routine for the last three months of pregnancy; there's no getting around that fact. The greatest comfort is that pregnancy doesn't go on forever. When my first child was small, we used to take long car rides to visit my family in the East. That was long before cars were outfitted with DVD players and other gadgets to amuse the children, and I sat with her in the back seat, trying to keep her happy. Every time we went through a tollbooth, she would say, "Are we there yet?" As she got older and could count, she would ask how many tollbooths were left until home. We couldn't tell her, because we didn't know. She kept up the questions, and the more she asked, the faster we wanted to get home. That's how I always felt toward the end of my pregnancies: are we there yet?

Starting in the third trimester, some of the toughest work of pregnancy begins, both physical and psychological. It's not a little "bump" anymore, but a full-fledged watermelon. That watermelon takes up most of your abdomen, and your vital organs suffer the consequences. Your stomach is pushed up against your diaphragm, which results in the reflux that many women experience, even when taking just a small sip of water. Your bladder is squished into much tighter quarters, and you must get up to pee every hour. If you sneeze, laugh, or cough, you'd better have an extra pair of underpants handy. By the end of the third trimester, sleep is elusive, and the thought of sleeping on your belly can rival the fantasy of winning a million dollars in the lottery.

While you are struggling with the physical aches and pains, new psychological fears may begin to arise: How will the baby get out? What if I can't do it? What if it hurts too much or I have to have a C-section? Will I embarrass myself by screaming too loudly or by losing control of my bowels in front of everyone? One way or another, the baby has to be delivered. There's no turning back, no changing your mind. Old worries also take on new intensity: Will the baby be healthy? Will I be a good mother?

For most women, pregnancy is joyful and tough, tougher particularly toward the end. The last four weeks seem to pass in slow motion. During the last weeks of my pregnancies, I imagine that no one could tolerate being around me. I couldn't tolerate being around myself. Every part of my body hurt, and the only way I could fall asleep was by wedging my huge self into a corner of the living room sofa. My emotions were on a roller coaster, and I would cry at nothing, frequently.

When Will This Be Over?

Darcey and I were having lunch at our favorite tearoom. My enormous belly was resting on my lap, and sweat was running down my legs. Being nine months' pregnant in August in

Houston is a challenge of enormous proportions. While taking a bite of a cucumber and cream cheese sandwich, I remarked to Darcey, "I don't think I can stand another day of this. They have got to get this baby out of me. There's a foot rammed up between my fifth and sixth ribs, and its head is grinding on my bladder." My eyes filled with tears. "I'm so tired and hot and cranky. I'm miserable."

Darcey, who is also a psychiatrist, always says just the right thing. "Sweetie, it's almost over, and then you'll have this adorable baby girl in your arms. I'll help you. Let's get moving and make the time go by. Tomorrow we'll book a pregnancy massage and a pedicure. I'll come pick you up."

I knew that she understood what I was feeling, and she knew that I needed some nurturing. The next day, it felt so good to have someone rub my aching back and to soak my swollen, tired feet in a warm whirlpool bath.

During the third trimester, it's important to take care of yourself both physically and emotionally. Being pregnant is hard work. Some women make it look easy, but for most of us, it's a demanding, intense job. And during the last several months, you often feel as if you're all tapped out.

Not only do you have the discomfort of carrying a large weight in your abdomen (and lower, as the weeks roll by), but you also have to deal with the emotions that rage through your body. By the end of your pregnancy, the levels of estrogen and progesterone coursing through your bloodstream are higher than they will ever be again. As I've already mentioned, these hormones, which promote the growth of the fetus, can have profound effects on your moods. During the third trimester, yet another hormone kicks in to help prepare your body for the birth. Relaxin begins its work of softening the cartilage in your joints so that the baby can get through your bony pelvis. Although this is a good thing, it is also responsible for the aches and pains you feel as your hips and pelvis widen and your ligaments stretch. It's an uncomfortable necessity.

Perhaps the biggest hurdle of the third trimester is the increasing feeling of vulnerability. Your belly no longer seems like a private part of your body. Strangers pat it and ask how soon the baby is due. They can't seem to help it. I was always amazed that anyone felt they had the right to touch my belly and then comment on how big or small I was when I told them my due date. At what other time in your life does the public at large feel it's okay to touch your body and then comment on your size? It's enough to keep you out of the supermarket or shopping mall. Nosy strangers aren't a huge problem, of course, but they are symbolic of the loss of autonomy you feel in the last months of pregnancy. This loss of autonomy also highlights the fact that you do need help. You simply can't meet all the obligations of ordinary life, no matter how much you want to. Many independent women don't want to be babied, but we all need to be nurtured and helped as pregnancy draws to a close.

I Can Do It Myself, Thank You

Millie was having trouble. I could see it in her face as she lumbered into my office. She had been crying, and she sat in that feet-on-the-floor, toes-and-knees-pointing-out position that women adopt in the last month of pregnancy in order to make room for the baby taking up all of their laps.

"I can't take it," she moaned. Her ankles were swollen, her back was hurting, she had to pee every fifteen minutes, around the clock, and nobody was helping her. Millie was nineteen years old and worked in a school cafeteria, so she was on her feet all day. She was trying to finish up her GED (general equivalency diploma) at night. Her husband, Martin, was working and attending college, so she had to do all the cooking and cleaning so that he could study for school.

Millie had dropped out of high school to marry Martin and had gone to work right away to help put him through college. Millie's parents had been unhappy with her decisions and had pulled away from the young couple. In response, Millie had set her shoulders and faced the world with determination and bravado. She would make it on her own without asking anyone for anything. And she was doing quite a job — full-time work, night classes, a house and husband to care for — until she found herself unexpectedly pregnant.

The bravado had departed, and Millie felt deflated; she couldn't do it alone, and she was still angry with her parents for their negative reaction. When she told her mother she was pregnant, there was no excitement, just a look that said, "I told you so." As for Martin, Millie didn't want to ask him to help. He was already doing all that he could to try to get ahead for their family.

"What would it take to call your mom?" I inquired.

Millie flushed and said, "I'm not going to do that." I looked at her inquiringly, and she continued, "I'm not going to admit I can't do it all myself. She would be too happy."

"Happy?" I asked.

Millie was imagining that her parents were just waiting for her to fail so that they could step in and take control of her life. They'd wanted Millie to stay in school and had offered to loan the young couple money so that she would only have to work after school. Millie had wanted to prove to them that she was a grownup and that she and Martin had made the right decision to marry. "I can do it myself," she'd told her parents, and she'd decided that she would never go to them for help. Asking for it now would be admitting defeat.

There was not much time to work with Millie, because the delivery was coming soon. I tried to help her see that being pregnant is hard on anyone, even the CEO of a Fortune 500 company, and that asking for help isn't a sign of weakness, but a sign of maturity. Going to her parents with a plan of how they could help would give her the relief she needed and show her mom that she wasn't a stubborn teenager anymore, but a young woman growing up. Independence is highly valued in our culture. For Millie, at this necessarily dependent time in her life, asking for help would be a sign of strength.

Millie finally did ask her mother for help, but set limits with her mother on how much control Millie was willing to give up. Millie's mother softened some as the delivery of her first grandchild approached and stopped being so critical. A beginning peace was created.

Birthing Plans

There are many physical demands during the third trimester: How do I get myself out of this chair? How do I pick up that shirt I dropped on the floor? How is this baby going to get out of me? Delivering the baby is a practical reality but also a psychological leap of faith. I've heard many intelligent women revert back to the voice of an eight-year-old who has just heard where babies come from: "That thing comes out of *where?* There's no way it's going to fit." Being reassured that babies have been coming out of vaginas for millennia does nothing to assuage the fear that a woman may feel when she imagines herself giving birth.

In chapter 2, I mentioned what I call the conspiracy of silence concerning the sharing of honest information with pregnant women. Unfortunately, there's too little silence when it comes to telling war stories at baby showers: "Oh, I was in labor for four days, and then finally the doctor gave me something for the pain." "After my baby was born, I was so torn up I couldn't sit down for a month. And going to the bathroom without screaming? Forget about it." Of course, there's always one who got it exactly right: "I've had three children, all of them naturally. Went back to work the following week in my size 6 blue jeans. Piece of cake." Why do we do that to one another?

Birthing plans have become a popular way of trying to help women have some control over what happens in the delivery room. They are often negotiated with the doctor or nurse practitioner ahead of time and usually entail much discussion between partners. Where should we have the baby, at home or in the hospital? Should we use a birthing room? What kind of music should we play? Do I want any kind of pain medication? What about sitting up on a birthing stool? Who should be in the delivery room with us? What about a nurse-midwife?

Some birthing plans are simple: "Get this baby out of me any way you can. Now." Others are more complicated: "Well, I'd really prefer that when the baby is born, there is soft lighting in the room. And I'm not fond of the idea of an episiotomy, if you don't mind."

A birthing plan starts with you and your partner discussing how you want the birth of your baby to go, then discussing your plan with your doctor. The hope is that you will be less likely to have to make an important decision in the midst of an excruciating contraction. Having a plan is not necessarily a bad idea, but it's important to realize that whether or not you accomplish your plan is not indicative of your value as a woman or a mother. A birthing plan can be a guideline for you and your health care provider to follow, but it may need to be changed at any moment for the safety and comfort of you and your baby.

Sometimes women compare their plans after the fact and discuss how closely they were able to follow them. The one who followed her plan exactly is deemed the victor. Those who had to give in to pain medication or a cesarean section feel diminished. Again, why do we do that to one another — and ourselves?

Is It My Hormones or Something More Serious?

One of the challenges I am sometimes faced with in my practice is trying to determine whether a woman is experiencing the normal mood fluctuations of late pregnancy caused by the enormous hormonal changes or is in the midst of something more serious that needs to be treated medically. But even if medication or therapy is not indicated, it's important to take these emotional issues seriously, for the sake of both the mother-to-be and those who love and care for her.

MY NEIGHBOR TOM knocked on my door late one night. "Could I have a minute of your time?" he asked. "There's a question I'd like to ask."

As a physician, I never know what those "minute of your time" encounters might entail. They can range from wanting me to look at a rash to asking me to stop the hemorrhaging from a kitchen knife accident. I've learned to be prepared for anything.

In this case, I knew that Tom's wife, Julie, was about to deliver their second child. Was he going to ask me to lend him a cup of sugar, or was the baby on its way? "Sure," I said, praying that it would be the former.

Tom looked at his feet and said, "It's just that Julie has been crying on and off since early this morning, and I'm not quite sure what to do. We got into a really big fight, and she told me to get out of the house. I wonder, do you have a sofa I could sleep on?"

Oh, my. This was not a stand-on-the-front-porch kind of conversation, nor did I want to invite him in to sleep on my sofa. Julie and I are iced tea–drinking neighbors: we occasionally sit on one of our porches and chat over a cold drink. I definitely didn't want to get in the middle of an argument between her and her husband.

I knew that she'd been struggling with the demands of a small child and another child on the way. I also knew that although Tom was doing his best, he was confused by Julie's mood changes from one minute to the next. My best guess was that he had reached his limit on patience, and that the fight had been the result.

After a brief exchange, I decided that the best approach would be to offer Tom a sit-down on our front porch with his own glass of tea while I went to check on Julie. I assumed that nothing much had changed since she and I had chatted the day before, but I wanted to be careful I wasn't missing something more serious. As expected, Julie was exhausted from lack of sleep, hurting all over, and feeling as if each day was a week. She needed sleep badly. In the lead-up to the fight, she'd wanted Tom to take their four-year-old for a while so that she could have some quiet time. Everything Tom said to her sounded like nails on a chalkboard. She needed him out of the house for a while, too, but knowing she felt that way had hurt his feelings.

She'd resorted to screaming at him, just to get him to go away. I left Julie with some suggestions for how she might sleep more comfortably and returned to sort things out with Tom.

I assured him that Julie was struggling with the normal moodiness of late pregnancy and certainly wasn't at her best. For a short while, I told him, he'd have to be extraordinarily patient with her and try to remember that her irritability had nothing to do with him. I also told him that the pregnancy was hard on him right now and that he needed to do something to relieve his own stress. Getting a sitter to take their child for an outing while Julie slept and he went out for a beer with the guys might be a great break for both of them. Armed with a new understanding and some time apart to deal with his own frustrations and worries, Tom went back and resolved the situation with Julie. They both thanked me later for helping them through a tough time.

It's not at all uncommon for a woman to cry at the drop of a hat during this time. (Commercials for Jell-O and puppy food were my particular weaknesses.) Estrogen and progesterone levels are approaching their highest peak and are responsible for the mood swings common at this stage of the pregnancy. A phone call at the wrong time or running out of salt can feel so overwhelming that the tears start to flow. The combination of fatigue, fear, and hormones can get the better of anyone. Irritability can rear its ugly head, and just a funny look from a loved one can start what feels like World War III. The important thing to remember is that this is all part of the last trimester, and no one should take the tears and the irritability personally.

❧

KIMBERLEY WAS IN her obstetrician's office begging to be delivered early. "I'm claustrophobic," she said. " I feel like the baby is taking up every inch of my body. I can't breathe, and I just want to run away from it all. I can't catch my breath. I feel like I'm going to panic. You have got to get this baby out of me *now*."

Her doctor tried to calm her down. "If we delivered your baby now, it would be far too early. He'd have to be in the intensive care nursery, and you don't want that. You're just going to have to wait it out. There's not that much time left."

Kimberley wasn't sure she could wait. In her mind, the baby had to be delivered now, or something bad was going to happen. She was having real anxiety and panic that needed to be treated with medication or relaxation therapy. Kimberley's situation was different from the typical frustrations and crankiness that can accompany the third trimester. Her symptoms were overpowering and interfering with her ability to function. She needed more serious help.

Pregnancy is a time of many emotions that change at the drop of a hat. But it is also a time when some women may experience more serious emotional symptoms that need to be treated.

In medical school in the 1980s, I was told that pregnancy protected women from developing psychiatric illness. I was taught that the high estrogen levels that occur during pregnancy keep women in a state of well-being, almost euphoria. Even today, some of my patients tell me that their psychiatrists advised them not to take their medication when they became pregnant because they would be feeling much better soon due to high estrogen levels. This is far from the truth.

Pregnancy does not prevent depression, anxiety, or any other psychiatric illness from occurring. Because many physicians were taught that pregnant women were protected during pregnancy, little attention was paid to the recognition and treatment of psychiatric symptoms during this time. Women who were pregnant were told that they could not take medication and were made to suffer until the baby was delivered. A pregnant woman has the same risk of becoming depressed as a woman who is not pregnant. The risk of psychiatric illness is greatest during the reproductive years, and becoming pregnant does not decrease this risk. In fact, one woman in four will have some type of depressive episode at some point during her lifetime. It stands to reason that some of those women will be pregnant when they become ill.

A physician would never consider not treating high blood pressure in a pregnant woman. The risk to the mother of untreated hypertension is great: heart disease, stroke, kidney problems. The risk to the fetus can be great as well: low birth weight, intrauterine stroke, placental abruption, and death. Even though the medications used to treat hypertension are not as well studied as psychiatric medications during pregnancy, physicians consider it necessary to control the mother's blood pressure. The same should be true for psychiatric medications.

If a pregnant woman doesn't need a medication, she shouldn't take it. This is true for all medications. Even if we know that a medication is perfectly safe during pregnancy, it does not make sense to expose the unborn baby to it if the benefit to the mother is insignificant.

The first question a physician needs to ask is, Do you need this medication to stay well? This question applies to any medication you might consider taking during pregnancy. To answer this question, you must consider how the illness started, what the symptoms were, how severe the symptoms were, and how long they lasted. Specifically in regard to psychiatric medications, the physician needs to ask, Did you ever need to be hospitalized in a psychiatric hospital? Have you ever attempted suicide or had serious thoughts of suicide that scared you? There is a big difference between a mild depression that does not cause much distress and an illness so severe that you are at serious risk for suicide or other harm.

The physician also should ask questions about your medication history — for instance, What is the longest period you have stayed well off medication? If it's been several years, you may be able to get through your pregnancy without medication and remain well. If, however, you quickly relapse when you go off medication, there is not much hope that you will be able to get through even the first trimester without it.

Supply your doctor with an accurate record of how many different medications you have been on, the dosages, and how well you responded to each. It is extremely helpful to have all this written down before you talk to your physician. If necessary, ask for records from your previous doctors so that you have a complete list. Although some medications may be preferred during pregnancy, if you have not responded well to them in the past, they are not an option. It is safer to stay on a medication that keeps you well than to switch to a "safer" medication that doesn't work for you.

Everyone involved should keep in mind that the decision about a particular medication must be made by the woman and her partner. Other physicians sometimes ask me what the best medication for, say, depression is for a woman during pregnancy. It is not that simple. Each patient is an individual; what may be right for one woman will not be right for another. My job is to ask the right questions, to provide information about the latest research, and to help the woman and her partner sort through their feelings. I can't make the decision for them.

If your child had an infection and penicillin was the only medication that would keep him alive, your doctor would be right to say, "We have to give your child this medication. There is nothing else to do. Without it, he will die." But deciding to use a psychiatric medication during pregnancy is not that clear-cut. The choices aren't black-and-white, and the outcome is uncertain. The couple, in collaboration with their physician, must decide what's best for them at the time.

I am often asked, "What would you do?" I have to reply, honestly, that I don't know. I don't know how bad someone feels and how much she is suffering. I don't know if she is able to function even though she's not feeling so great. I can't take into account what amount of risk to herself or her baby she is willing to tolerate. Some women are unable to tolerate any risk. They tell me, "I can't take medication. If something goes wrong, I will never be able to forgive myself. Even if it were due to some other reason, I would always blame the medication." These women need the highest standard of information available and will go to great lengths to obtain as much information as possible from every conceivable source. Other women are willing to tolerate at least a small amount of risk and are comfortable not knowing with absolute certainty that everything will be fine.

The woman's personal degree of comfort with the unknown needs to be factored into these decisions. I am not a big risk taker but can tolerate some risk. I begrudgingly fly, knowing it is possible, but highly unlikely, that the plane will crash. I am willing to tolerate a small degree of risk so that I can get from Houston to New York City without spending several days in a cramped car. Other people are much more comfortable with uncertainty and can tolerate a higher degree of risk; they will voluntarily hurl their bodies out of an airplane for the exquisite physical thrill and are willing to trust in parachute technology. Not me.

It's a Family Decision

A pregnant woman who needs an antidepressant or another psychiatric medication is often made to feel that she is doing something horrible to her unborn child. Pregnant women who need a psychiatric medication often suffer tremendously due to the stigma of mental illness. A woman's family, her spouse, and even her physician may believe that she should be able to "tough it out," that if she were a good mother, she would do anything not to harm her child. Some pregnant women are told that if they wish to continue to be treated by their obstetricians or their psychiatrists, they must stop taking a medication that keeps them well.

❧

BARBARA HAD SUFFERED from depression for many years. Her parents had divorced when she was young, and she had been shuttled back and forth between their homes. Several stepmothers and stepfathers had appeared and disappeared through the years. Inevitably, Barbara would get close to one, and then he or she would leave and quickly be replaced by another. As a result, she'd learned to shut the door on her emotions, and she spent much of her time alone in her room drawing.

Barbara did well in school and left home to attend a prestigious art program. At first she felt as if she was finally leaving her past behind and had the chance to start over. Unfortunately, at the age of eighteen she developed a severe depression that landed her in the hospital. It wasn't surprising, given all of the losses early in her life, that she would experience depression. She was placed on antidepressant medication and started therapy.

Barbara was lucky to find a therapist who nurtured her and

allowed her to feel loved and valued. This enabled her to see herself for the first time as a successful, worthwhile woman whom someone might be able to love. She dated a man she met in college, and they married shortly after graduation. Barbara remained in therapy and on medication for several years with good results. She occasionally felt down, but nothing like what had sent her to the hospital several years earlier. She and her husband felt that it was time to start a family.

Barbara was told by her psychiatrist that she would need to stop all of her medication prior to becoming pregnant. He told her that staying on the medication was not an option and that he would not continue to treat her if she took the medication while she was pregnant. Barbara and her husband were anxious not to do anything that might be harmful to their baby, so she abruptly stopped her medication and began trying to conceive.

"I started to feel bad almost immediately," she said. "I was crying all the time and felt as if I was totally out of control. We tried for over a year to get pregnant, but it just wasn't happening, and I was getting more and more depressed. I was so scared that I'd have to go into the hospital again. I finally got pregnant but was still miserable. After six months, I finally begged my doctor to put me back on my meds. He referred me to someone else, who agreed to treat me. But I was terrified the whole time something would be wrong with the baby."

What could have been a pleasurable experience turned into a nightmare for Barbara. Although she and her husband had talked about having a big family, she couldn't imagine ever having another child if it meant feeling that bad again. She felt terribly sad that having more children didn't seem to be an option for them.

I meet with women like Barbara every week. They have been told that taking psychiatric medication while pregnant is not an option, and yet they are afraid to stop taking it. Some women consider having an abortion because the baby has been exposed to psychiatric medication. Some reproductive endocrinologists won't attempt in vitro fertilization in a woman who is taking psychiatric medication — even when there is no evidence that the medication impairs fertility. Couples are torn between a desperate longing for children and the fear that the woman might become seriously ill if she stopped her medication. This is not a decision the woman can make by herself. Many people will have an opinion about her decision.

SUSAN WAS TWENTY-FIVE and near the end of her first pregnancy. Her husband, a family practice doctor, had kept a watchful eye on her. During her sixth month, she became very tearful, crying for no reason. She started to have trouble eating and sleeping. When she went to her obstetrician for a routine exam, she discovered that she had lost three pounds in the past month. When her obstetrician asked her how she was feeling, she began to cry. She told him that she was having serious doubts about having a baby and wasn't sure she could do it. Her doctor referred her to me after recommending that she start taking medication for her anxiety. She was scared to take medication while she was pregnant, and her husband was adamantly opposed to it.

Susan asked if she could bring her husband, Louis, to her first appointment. I said of course. It is pointless for me to counsel a woman alone if there is someone else involved who will have an influence on the decision she makes. I want to have the chance to answer everyone's questions and clear up any misperceptions. I've had as many as five people in my office at one time, all asking questions and voicing opinions about what was best for the mother-to-be. Similarly, I've seen many women decide it was time to take a medication but then change their minds after telling their families and receiving strong negative reactions. It is hard to go against so much negativity when you are feeling scared and overwhelmed.

I spent an hour with Susan and Louis, asking questions about Susan's symptoms and explaining the options to them. It was clear to me that Susan was having moderately severe symptoms of anxiety and depression and needed medication. One of her statements concerned me. She said, "I feel so anxious and upset. I don't know what I'm going to do. I think about being with a new baby, and I just don't think I can handle it. The other day I was driving, and I had to pull over to the side of the road. I was hyperventilating, and my heart was pounding. I just kept thinking about driving off a bridge and ending it all."

"How serious are those thoughts?" I asked. "Do they scare you?" I get very anxious when I hear words like Susan's. Often it is just a thought or a feeling that the woman has no intention of acting on. That's okay. When someone is depressed, the wish to escape the sadness and hopelessness is not uncommon. At other times, however, expressing such thoughts is more serious and may actually be the beginning of a plan to carry them out. I always ask. Not to ask invites tragedy.

"Well, I know I won't do anything to hurt myself, but I'm just so miserable," Susan said. "I don't know what to do. Sometimes I think it would be easier if I weren't here, but I know that's crazy. Do you think these feelings are just because I'm pregnant? I've heard that women become very emotional toward the end. I think I'm making too big a deal out of things. Maybe I'm just having normal pregnancy worries."

I told her that her thoughts and feelings were way out of proportion with what would be considered normal. Worries and anxieties about one's ability to mother are very common, but thoughts that it would be easier to go to sleep and not wake up are not. Those symptoms need to be treated. I turned to Louis and asked him what he was thinking.

"I haven't noticed that there was anything wrong," he said. "She's been a little tearful, but I've seen a lot of pregnant women who get moody toward the end of their pregnancy. We are really against her taking any medication while she is pregnant. I mean, I get depressed and anxious sometimes, and then I just get over it. I don't need to take medication. Everyone gets that way sometimes."

This is a common response from someone who has never experienced the symptoms of clinical depression or anxiety. Everyone gets "depressed" sometimes and may even wonder if life's worth living. But a true medical depression is a very different experience. The feelings and symptoms don't go away quickly. They last for a long time and are present most of the time on an almost daily basis. It's not something you can "get over." No matter how hard you try to talk yourself out of it or make sense of it, you can't by sheer force of will make the feelings go away.

I explained to Louis that I believed Susan was struggling with something very different from just "feeling down." She needed treatment. I turned to her and said, "How do you feel about starting medication?"

"Well, I usually depend on Louis to help me make medical decisions. But to be fair, I really haven't told him how bad I've been feeling. I thought maybe it would go away and that I was overreacting to being pregnant. I've been trying to hide how miserable I am from him. I guess if you think I need medication, maybe I do. I don't know. What do you think, Louis?" Without waiting for an answer, she turned to me and said, "If he's against it, I don't want to take anything. I'd feel so guilty if anything went wrong."

To his credit, Louis said that if I thought she would do better on medication, they could try it and see. He wanted to do what was best for Susan and the baby. He didn't really understand what she was going through, and maybe he never would.

I started Susan on an antidepressant that would treat both her depressive and her anxiety symptoms. She called me three weeks later to tell me how much better she was feeling. She continued to do well for the rest of her pregnancy. I got a phone call from her when the baby was two weeks old. Everything was "great," she said, and she was enjoying being a new mom.

Psychiatric illness has nothing to do with strength or weakness, goodness or badness. Psychiatric illness is like any other medical disorder. Pregnant women are treated daily for asthma, diabetes, high blood pressure, even cancer. No one makes them feel guilty about having these disorders. Everyone understands that illness is often beyond a person's control. It is a matter of genetics, environmental factors, or even just plain bad luck. Psychiatric disorders are no different than physical ones.

It is important that a pregnant woman is given the support she needs not only to deliver a healthy baby but also to ensure that the baby has a healthy mother. If you decide that taking medication is the right decision for you, make sure that the physicians you see are supportive. It is always a good idea for your obstetrician and the baby's pediatrician to be included in the decision-making process. They need to know what the plan is and agree to it. Your pediatrician and obstetrician should have your baby's and your best interests at heart.

Sometimes it may be necessary to change doctors if your physician is unable to support you in these decisions. I refer patients to several obstetricians who have made it a point to understand psychiatric illness and medication. They are willing to work with pregnant women to help them make the best decisions. We work closely together to ensure the best possible outcome for both mother and baby.

· TIPS ·

1. *Putting your needs first.* This is a time when you need to be sure that you are taking care of yourself and not trying to prove something to yourself, your family, or the world. Choose the pampering techniques that work for you: special teas that you love, a weekly date at the nail parlor, massages, or time spent with people who will nurture you.

If your maternity clothes are getting tight or you can't stand putting on the same two maternity tops every other day, get yourself to the store one last time. It may seem silly to buy a new outfit when there's only a month or so left, but having something new to wear that fits and makes you feel less enormous may help your outlook and your mood.

If you are tired, go to bed. It's important to sleep whenever you can. You may not be able to sleep for several hours in a row, but intermittent sleep is better than no sleep. When every position you try puts pressure on some part of you, try using a body pillow. It can make the difference between a restful night's sleep and pacing the floor trying to find a place to get comfortable. Sleeping in a recliner can support your back, elevate your feet, and allow you to be in a comfortable position other than on your side. You may miss cuddling with your partner in bed, but at this stage of the pregnancy, sleep is of primary importance.

2. *The baby shower.* It is time to take control of the traditional baby shower. Showers can be lots of fun and a great way to stock your nursery with necessary and pricey items. But showers where you open box after box of adorable (and expensive) baby clothes are a waste of time and money. Many of the clothes you receive

never fit, are never worn, or are stained with breast milk or vomit five minutes after you put them on the baby. I'm not against beautiful clothes, but there are so many other things that can be more beneficial to a new mother.

If family and friends ask you about a shower, consider offering these suggestions. How about a "shower" of meals, baby-sitting older children, or doing the laundry? I attended one shower where the woman's coworkers organized two weeks of home-cooked meals delivered to her home after her baby was born. What a relief not to have to worry about how to feed yourself and your family while you're also trying to learn to breastfeed. Or how about gifts of time — sitting with the new baby (or older children) while you have your hair cut, go for a massage, or just take a walk or sit on the front porch? Being able to get out of the house for even a short while can feel like the greatest gift of all. So let Grandma buy the frilly cute clothes and ask for something you can use to start your lives together well fed and well rested.

3. *Your postpartum plan.* Planning for the arrival of your new baby may be the most important task of the third trimester. Having a well-thought-out plan (see the appendix) will help decrease the sense of being overwhelmed when the nurse puts the baby in your arms and you realize this new little person is going home with you. It also will minimize your risk of developing anxiety and depression. Your plan should include not just what color the nursery will be or what kind of car seat you will buy for the ride home. More important issues include the following: What kind of help will you need when you get home? Who will come to visit and when? Will your husband take off work during the first week, or will he wait until later? How will you make sure you get enough sleep? Who will watch the other children so that they don't become bored or resentful of the new

baby? Who will prepare the meals and do the laundry those first few weeks?

For some women, the answer to these questions is easy: Mom, of course. Some new grandmothers go into superwoman mode when there is a new baby in the house. They cook, clean, do laundry, and get up with the baby in the middle of the night. But not every woman is so lucky, or this plan may not work for you. If, for example, you don't have a good relationship with your mother or mother-in-law, immediately after the birth might not be the best time for her to visit. A newborn will stress even the healthiest relationship, let alone one where there is already resentment or hurt feelings. In these cases, ask your mother or mother-in-law to come when the baby is four to six weeks old. You will feel physically better and have a better handle on how to care for your baby. Tell her you want her to come when you'll be more settled and have more time to enjoy her visit. If she insists on coming immediately after the baby is born, explain that you have a plan for who will be helping when and ask her to honor that. She's welcome to come, but when you and your baby come home from the hospital, *your* needs must take priority.

Do not schedule all of your help to come for the first two weeks. Many new mothers have described to me the total terror they felt when all of the relatives went home and they were alone. You go from having too many hands to having none. Ask your mother to come the first week, your mother-in-law the second, your sister the third, and your best friend from Albuquerque the fourth. They will enjoy not having to compete with one another to hold the baby and will have more of your attention. You will enjoy not being overwhelmed with company and will be glad to have the help spread out over a longer period of time. By the end of the fourth week, you should be feeling much more confident in your role as a new mother.

Some new families decide that they want to get used to the new baby without outside interference during the first week. This can work well as long as your partner understands that you will need a lot of help. Other families decide to wait until all the relatives have gone home for the father to take time off from work. That way, he can be with his new family after things have calmed down. It might not make sense for Dad to take time off when there is other help available and he will be competing with them to be part of the team.

$$5$$

The Big Day

The big day is coming. Your due date is near; the baby is showing signs of being ready to be born; the doctor says everything is on schedule. But nobody knows exactly when labor will begin, and there may be many false starts before the baby actually arrives.

Waiting for labor to begin is for many women a profound lesson in patience. Somehow, even though the doctors and all the experts tell us that the due date is an approximation, women hold that day in their heads like a mantra. Everyone in the family is impatient for labor to start. Numerous phone calls are made to ask if anything has happened yet. It's hard for a nine-months'-pregnant woman to sleep, and every little twinge takes on unnerving significance. And, at least for the first week or so after the due date has passed, there's nothing to do but wait.

Some women don't do well with waiting. While my friend Jane was waiting, she rode into New York City with her husband on his daily commute so that she could ride the subway. It didn't help. She walked; she jumped. It didn't help. When she turned up at the doctor's office for her second post–due date appointment, the nurse who had been her best buddy for (more than) nine months saw her and said, "You still here?" Jane had heard that too many times, and she broke down in tears. Nature eventually took its course, but for Jane, as for many women, the waiting was excruciating.

The last few weeks of pregnancy are an extraordinary mix of excitement, fatigue, anxiety, and joy. It's hard to believe that this long trip is almost over. Trouble sleeping, being pummeled in the ribs and bladder by the baby's knees and elbows, swollen feet and hands — all these will be over after the baby is delivered. But even with the many techniques of diagnosing problems ahead of time, and being fairly certain the baby has the correct number of fingers and toes, there is still the fear of the unknown. What if something goes wrong? What if a genetic problem was missed? It's only when they hear that first cry and can count ten fingers and toes that most women breathe a sigh of relief.

Since time immemorial, women have delivered their young, but still the task seems overwhelming. It's nearly impossible to imagine getting a life-size newborn out of your body. "Can I do this?" you wonder. "What if I fail?" One way to assuage your fears is to attend Lamaze classes, so that you can practice breathing and become something of an expert on the process of giving birth. These things, along with a tour of the hospital and conversations with doctors and midwives, will help you devise a plan, which in turn will help you deal with some prebirth anxiety.

There is only one problem with planning: you have to be sure that you aren't setting yourself up for disappointment or a sense of failure. Every woman is different, and so is every labor. If you judge yourself a success or failure according to a plan made weeks or months ahead, you may be headed for trouble. Instead, make this your motto: Expect the unexpected.

Sometimes a baby comes early, before the baby shower and the last Lamaze class. Women whose babies arrive early may mourn the loss of that final week or two of pregnancy and the special plans they had for that time. They'll have to deal with thrown-together nurseries and hand-me-down baby clothes for a while.

Some women who were ready to withstand the pain of labor without medication find themselves asking for help very soon. Others don't understand what all the fuss was about. Just to make things more complicated, a woman's second or third delivery may be totally different from her first. How you deal with these uncertainties and differences has a lot to do with your experience of childbirth.

Since everything is unpredictable — from when labor will start to how long it will take to how hard (or easy) it will be — you'll need help in adopting a "what will be, will be" attitude. I know that's much easier said than done, and you'll need all the reassurance you can get so that you are not disappointed and won't take unreasonable responsibility if there are problems. It's not your fault if your water breaks when you're in a cab with your boss or you have three false starts. It's not your fault if the baby comes in the car or labor takes thirty-six hours. It's not your problem if you can't keep your husband from fainting or yelling at the doctor, or if you can't prevent your in-laws from acting up at the hospital. Giving birth is a time of supreme effort. It's what has kept the human race alive for millions of years. It's not a ballet performance or a final exam. You are the heroine of this story, no matter what you yell, how you behave, or what you say to the doctor. Believe me, other women — plenty of them — have been much worse.

For some women, the act of giving birth is a wonderful experience, and everything goes as planned. The pregnancy is easy, labor and delivery are a piece of cake, and the baby is healthy and beautiful. But much more often, there are disappointments and readjustments. Even so, with the next pregnancy, it's hard not to hope that *this* time the delivery will turn out just as planned.

For the birth of my first child, I planned an idyllic delivery in a birthing suite, complete with soft lighting, a rocking chair, and a soothing whirlpool bath. At that time, hospital policy was that a woman could be in the birthing room only if she wasn't going to use medication to control pain. If she needed medication, she was moved into a labor room and then wheeled into the delivery room for the actual birth. (The delivery room was outfitted as an operating room; it was the same place where cesarean sections were performed.) So just as the woman was about to push her baby out, she would be transferred to a gurney and rushed, moaning, down the hall to the delivery room. Fortunately, birthing practices have changed over the years.

Never having delivered a baby before, I assumed that I could handle the pain. I had taken birthing classes, had learned self-hypnosis techniques, and had a husband who was going to stand by my side the whole time. After about forty-five minutes of hard labor, however, I started to panic. It hurt like hell. I asked the nurse to check my progress, and she told me that I was dilated to two centimeters and probably had many more hours to go until I was fully dilated to ten. I looked at my husband and saw fear in his eyes. We do have one very nice picture of me taken in the birthing room: I'm smiling as a nurse checks my belly for the fetal heart tones. The rest is a blur, although I recall being in the delivery room and begging to be put to sleep.

Child number four: I refused to give up. "Okay, I admit I

cursed at the obstetrician last time, but she was ordering take-out from the delivery room. It was hard to take that my competition was an order of crispy fried chicken. I really think I have it in me this time." I wanted the perfect birth experience. I knew this was absolutely going to be my last child, and I wanted to do it my way.

Skepticism notwithstanding, my husband agreed to give it another go-round. This time I would be armed not only with panting but also with soothing music, a peaceful focal point, and a new obstetrician who understood how important it was for me not to have my feet up in stirrups when the baby came out. (We'd discussed how the need for an episiotomy may be much less if you can labor in an upright squatting position.) I was desperate to get it right on try number four.

Everything started as anticipated. I was wearing my comfortable pajamas, my favorite nurse was on duty (they knew me in labor and delivery; I was famous for that fried chicken incident), and the perfect birthing music was playing on my boom box. Things went really well for about the first twenty minutes. Lots of expert breathing and some really great lower back rubs compliments of my sweet husband. And then my water broke. The rupturing of the amniotic membranes is a pivotal moment in any labor process. At that point, the baby's head begins to pound directly on the cervix without the benefit of a nice watery cushion. I began to scream for an epidural.

"Now, honey," my husband reminded me, "you said if you started to scream for pain meds, I was supposed to ignore you. Do you really want them, or should I pretend I didn't hear you? Here, concentrate on the soothing sounds of the ocean." He held the boom box closer to my ear. At that moment, the supposedly dulcet cawing of the seagulls interrupted the soothing sound of crashing waves. I looked at him with evil intent and threw the boom box across the room. "Get rid of the damn seagulls," I said. "I can't take them."

"Okay, honey, then let's try some James Taylor," my suddenly infuriating husband said. I love James Taylor. I have loved his music since I was seventeen years old and had my dorm room walls papered with his adorable face. But at that moment, "Sweet Baby James" was not going to do anything to distract me from the inexorable efforts of a very large baby trying to squeeze through a very small opening. I caved in.

"I want pain meds, and I want them now. I don't care who gives them to me, how they get here, or where they come from, but if the anesthesiologist doesn't get here immediately, I will sue everyone in this entire hospital." In another twenty minutes, I was smiling, pain-free, and playing a round of poker with the night staff. My befuddled husband sat in the corner wondering where he'd gone wrong.

Four hours later, we had a beautiful, very large baby girl, and my tubes were tied. My dreams of the "perfect" delivery were over — and it made absolutely no difference at all. I had a sweet new daughter, and I loved her. I suffered for a few weeks with a sore bottom but let go of the idea that somehow I had failed by not delivering a baby the "right" way. I did it the way I needed to and the best way I could at the time.

Sometimes things are out of your control. You shouldn't feel awful if you hoped for a natural delivery but ended up with a cesarean section; if you hoped for no meds but ended up with an epidural or other pain medication; if you hoped for serenity but ended up throwing your boom box across the room.

Giving birth to a child isn't a performance; it is a difficult and taxing job. Women's fears and unreasonable expectations of themselves can only make this job harder. We need to dispel the myths about labor and delivery and to help women be more accepting of themselves throughout this process.

Bonding

Women are told by television, books, and other mothers that giving birth is one of the most important and fulfilling things they can do and that they should be ecstatic from the first moment the baby is laid naked at their breast. The "ideal" experience is that the child will be placed on your abdomen immediately after it is pulled from you, cord still attached. At that moment, the fairy tale goes, you are overcome by a blissful feeling, a fierce connection of love. The baby opens his eyes to gaze into yours, and it's a match made in heaven. In one extraordinary film that I was shown during my psychiatry residency, the baby, ready to nurse, began to attempt to squirm upward to the waiting breast.

We are told that bonding occurs in that split second and that lifelong connections and attachments are formed. We are also told that if this process is interrupted, mother and child will never be whole. That is a huge expectation, and it is simply not true.

But women worry. What happens if this exquisite connection at birth doesn't occur? What if my baby is ill and needs immediate medical attention? What if I glance down at the baby and am just thankful that it's finally out of my body? Very often a new mother looks at the squished little creature (not all newborns look like cherubs) and is stunned by the lack of recognition and feeling. Particularly if a woman received pain medication during childbirth, both she and her baby may be feeling dazed and exhausted. In some instances, the attachment can take weeks or even months to form. These mothers ask me if there is something wrong with them because they weren't immediately in love with their babies. Of course there is nothing wrong with them. Some people take time to warm up to a newborn. In fact, a lot of people prefer older babies, even toddlers.

You *will* grow to love your baby over time. The wonderful thing is that infants are programmed to be adorable, to attract love and attention. That's a survival tactic, built into the DNA to ensure that babies are fed and properly cared for. Infant smells and behaviors go a long way toward making parents fall in love with them. But it's not always love at first sight.

I'm not saying this doesn't ever happen. It didn't for me, but I have spoken to other mothers who described their overwhelming feelings of love and joy once their babies were placed on their bellies. I have also heard from new moms who didn't have those feelings for several weeks or months. "Is there something wrong with me?" they ask. "Am I a bad mother?"

❦

STEPHANIE LABORED FOR eighteen hours and was exhausted. "I couldn't imagine they would ever get the baby out," she said. "I pushed for over two hours and wasn't making any progress at all. The baby was face-up, not face-down, so it wasn't going as smoothly as it was supposed to. And then the doctor mentioned forceps."

Forceps look like salad tongs. They are designed to wrap around the baby's head and to help pull it past the pubic bones and into the world. If the procedure is done carefully, mother and baby do just fine. It is often used as a way to avoid a cesarean section or to get the baby out quickly if there is some distress. But the experience can be somewhat physically and psychologically traumatic. It can be scary to think of your baby being pulled out of you with large metal salad tongs.

"All I remember about the delivery is how tired I was and how grateful I was that it was finished," Stephanie said. "When they put Grant up on my stomach, I didn't feel anything — just relief. I mean, I was happy and all, but I didn't feel this connection everybody talks about. Do you think it's too late to bond? Will he and I ever be close?"

Childbirth is a demanding job that takes stamina, perseverance, and patience. It's also exciting and frightening. Your body has started a process that can't be stopped, and there's no time-out, no "Let me come back another day; I changed my mind." For some women, labor can be fast and easy, but that's the exception. For most of us, it is the most demanding physical experience we will ever undertake. Once the baby is born, it takes our bodies and minds several hours, days, and weeks to incorporate that overwhelming and emotional event.

After delivering a baby, you face competing needs: the need to rest; to finally have something to eat and drink; to wrap your mind around what just happened to you. And then there's the baby. You might think, "What do I do now? I'm tired, yet I'm supposed to be breastfeeding on demand. I want to talk to my best friend, but there is an endless stream of visitors at the door bringing food and flowers. I don't want my other children to feel left out, but I want to snuggle with my sweet new baby."

My friend Halley tells the story of sitting in her hospital bed, ten hours after her first daughter was born. The baby was squalling, and she couldn't figure out how to nurse. She couldn't calm the baby either. Halley was about to fall apart when she looked down at the squirming, bawling baby and said, "We don't know each other yet, but we're going to be together for a long time. I'll try my best, and I know you'll do the same. We'll get through it somehow." Halley was a little calmer after her speech to the newborn, and so was the baby, who is now a college graduate. Halley has repeated these words to her child many times, and they have helped mother and daughter through many crises.

❧

MARIA HAD AN easy labor and pushed for only forty-five minutes before her beautiful baby girl was born. But when the baby didn't cry, Maria saw everyone in the room rushing around and heard them speaking in quiet yet insistent voices. The next thing Maria and her husband, Fred, knew, the nurses had rushed the baby out of the birthing room and down the hall to the special care nursery.

This wasn't what they had planned. Maria was lying with her feet in the stirrups while her obstetrician sewed up the episiotomy. Her baby was nowhere to be seen. She had imagined her baby lying in her arms while Fred busily took digital pictures to send to friends and family. She had read how important it was for the baby to nurse as soon as it was born. That would start off a cascade of events that would ensure bonding and start mother and child down the path of connection and security. How was that going to happen when the baby was in a cold, sterile nursery?

Frantically, she sent Fred to the nursery to check on the baby. There were so many things going on that frightened her, but she was flat on her back, unable to move. It felt like hours before everyone left and she was alone. The first thing Maria did was call her sister, who had two children herself and had been very helpful during the pregnancy. She would know how to fix things.

Maria immediately started crying. "Something's wrong with the baby, and they took her away," she told her sister. "I didn't get to do anything I planned on. I'm so afraid that I'm missing out on everything. We'll never get this time back, and I'm afraid I won't get to bond. What if she doesn't attach to me or we can't learn how to breastfeed?"

Maria's baby had an infection and needed to stay in intensive care for a week while being treated with intravenous antibiotics. It was hard for Maria to get physically close to her baby, and more difficult still to see her beautiful newborn hooked up to tubes and machines. But the baby did well, and Maria remembers with great clarity the first time they put her daughter in her arms. "It no longer mattered that those first few days were a blur. The minute I put my face up to hers and she opened her eyes, I knew all was right with the world again. I was so overwhelmed with love and fear for her, I knew without a doubt I was her mother; and I would give up my life to protect her."

Many things may interfere with those idyllic first moments we all imagine, but the ties that bind mother and child together are not easily broken, even if "bonding" doesn't happen immediately.

Right-Away Emotions

The act of giving birth is one of the most creative and demanding things a person can do. Sometimes endorphins that were released during the work of labor leave mothers with a feeling of exaltation — a high that some women liken to a drug high. Feeling on top of the world, gathering congratulations from everybody, checking with your partner for the color of her eyes or whose mother she looks like, and joining the great chain of human life — all these can be thrilling. Other women are tired and ready to turn over and take a nap. That's great, too. Some women want to hold the baby until they are checked out of the hospital. Others want to leave the baby in the nursery until the car arrives in the hospital parking lot to take them home. Both reactions are fine.

After delivery, a radical shift in a woman's hormones begins, as the body begins to shrink the uterus and prepare for lactation. Estrogen and progesterone levels fall and oxytocin and prolactin are released to promote breastfeeding. Equally profound emotional changes can occur as well. Some women who were delighted with the prospect of impending parenthood, had perfectly acceptable labor, and delivered healthy babies find themselves unable to stop crying a few hours after delivery. A woman I know recounts the birth of her first child this way: "It all went fine. And let me tell you, we wanted this baby more than anything in the world. But when I finally got into my room after the baby was born, I started to cry as if my best friend had just died. I cried for hours. At one point, a pediatric resident walked into the room to check on the baby. When he saw me, he literally backed out of the room!"

The tears were gone after a few hours of sleep and a good breakfast. Although it wasn't funny at the time, we were able to laugh later at the thought of the young doctor actually being afraid of the crying new mother. She and I have six kids between us, and we both know that tears after childbirth are just part of the process.

The Circle of Life

The human world is made up of an amazing variety of people, and every parent has her or his own way of loving a child. Just as every parent is different, every baby is different — it's not just the fingerprints and footprints that vary. Some are alert from the beginning; others are too alert and seem to startle at the slightest noise. Some babies are placid and easy to calm; others seem almost too placid, and the new parents worry because of that. Most newborns look funny, especially if labor has been long and hard. They may have cone-shaped heads or swollen, lopsided features. That's the way it is. Cone-shaped heads round out, and swollen features diminish in size. Red skin turns pink, and skinny, scrawny babies become plump angels. First impressions and early moments are just that. There's no way of telling what kind of person your baby will grow up to be based on those first impressions. And there is no way to evaluate the kind of mother you are going to be from the experience of labor and childbirth.

Each of us has strengths and weaknesses. I'm really great with babies and teenagers. Go figure. But with kids between the ages of three and twelve, I lose my patience and equanimity. There's something about the endless, repetitive questions and desire to play games that doesn't lean into my strengths. Give me a crying baby or a petulant teenager, and I'm good to go. But playing even five minutes of Candy Land or speculating for the nineteenth time about why the grass is green makes me want to shut myself in my room for the next five or six years.

During those middle years, though, I'm still a good mother. Not the most pleasurable ages for me, but I can put my own needs on hold for a while and make it halfway through a game of cards. And I can manage to answer the green grass question one or two times. I'm able to give my kids love and consistency, and they know that I will be available to them when they need me. You will discover your own strengths and weaknesses as a parent — but not all at once; it will take time.

Giving birth is a miracle. The very act of giving birth makes you a hero. It doesn't matter if you hissed obscenities at your husband or the doctor; it doesn't matter if you asked for anesthesia when you promised not to; it doesn't matter if you had a C-section; it doesn't matter if you didn't fall immediately in love with your baby. If you are fortunate enough to get through the process of delivery and bring a new life into the world, you have succeeded.

· TIPS ·

1. *Waiting for baby.* The last several weeks of pregnancy can feel like forever. Each day seems endless; the physical discomforts magnify the slow passage of time. Focusing on every twinge or cramp that doesn't end in labor can be disheartening and frustrating.

Now is the time to stay distracted. Catch up on the movies you won't get to see once the baby arrives. If your doctor allows it, make sure you get some exercise every day. This will make you feel better and may encourage labor. Knitting or crocheting something for the baby to wear home from the hospital can be a good way to pass the time, and you will enjoy imagining the baby wearing it. If you feel up to it, prepare some meals for the freezer for after the delivery. These activities can make you feel as if you're accomplishing something, even if it's not labor.

If you're still working, staying busy may be easier than if you're sitting at home waiting. But working moms may have trouble staying focused on work, wondering every day, "Will I be here tomorrow?" It is best to be prepared to leave work at least two weeks before your due date. Have loose ends wrapped up and know who's going to be taking over your responsibilities. Make sure you've left instructions for what needs to be done if you go into labor early. If it's financially feasible, it may be nice to take at least one week off before the baby is expected. You may want some time to enjoy getting things ready at home. If, however, your maternity leave feels short, you may not want to use it up by taking time off before the baby is born.

Friends and relatives who are just as anxious as you are may not hesitate to call several times a day, asking, "Is there a baby yet?" The answer is of course not; otherwise you would have called them. Make an e-mail list and send out a daily bulletin on how you're feeling. Include the latest news from the doctor. Reassure family and friends that you will let them know as soon as there is news. Some couples put a message on the answering machine: "No baby yet — we'll let you know." Although this may not deter anxious grandmothers, it will slow down some others, who will be satisfied to wish you well by answering machine.

2. *Make the delivery yours.* The baby *will* come, and your body *will* do its job. It might not cooperate in the way you'd like it to — you may have a very painful labor or even need a C-section — but 95 percent of the women I talk to care very little about how the baby was born once the delivery is over. The pleasure of having the baby out of your body and finally getting to see the face of the person you've been carrying around all these months erases most memories of how difficult or disappointing the delivery might have been.

Before you go to the hospital, make sure you know whom you want in the delivery room with you and whom you want in the waiting room. Many things are out of your control, but who is in the room at this most intimate moment is entirely up to you. Don't wait until you're in labor to decide; you'll be too distracted to think straight. Some women want as many people as possible watching the new baby's arrival. Others want only their partners there. There is no right or wrong answer to this. Only you know what's comfortable for you.

Don't argue with your doctor about what is best for you. If you've been comfortable with your doctor this far, trust that she is continuing to put you and your baby's health at the forefront. If your doctor says you've labored too long and it's time to consider a C-section, she is thinking about the risks of prolonged labor. Don't be disappointed; your baby will be here much sooner and will be healthy. Don't, however, be afraid to ask why. You are allowed to know why certain things are happening to you. If you're not sure about what's being suggested, ask whether there is another option that also will ensure a healthy delivery. Some things may be set up for the doctor's comfort or convenience. Although this is important, your doctor may be willing to consider another way of doing things.

Bring pillows from home. Hospital pillows are notoriously uncomfortable, and it will be reassuring to be surrounded by your own comfortable bedding. Also bring a robe and slippers. It's nice to have a pretty robe to put on over your hospital gown. You'll also likely be walking the hospital hallways, and you'll definitely want to have something on your feet. Avoid packing fancy pajamas. You'll probably want to wear a hospital gown, which is made to get messy.

Take pictures and video. Believe it or not, the delivery may eventually become a blur, and you'll be glad you have a photographic record of this extraordinary event. Kids love looking at pictures of themselves right after they've popped out of Mom's tummy.

3. *The first few hours.* You will have many years to fall in love with your baby; don't overvalue the first few hours of your life together. If you feel great, then by all means keep the baby in your room as long as you like. Try breastfeeding, but remember that most babies — just like their mothers — need to learn how.

Turn off the phone, put a NO VISITORS sign on the door, and turn off the lights. You may be too wired to sleep for the first few hours after your baby is born, but sleep is imperative. At least the first night, let the baby spend a few hours in the nursery so that you can rest. The nursing staff will bring the baby to you when it's time to feed. There is no need to feel guilty about letting the baby stay in the nursery. You, too, are a patient and need time to recover. At this time, getting rehydrated, renourished, and rested will go far toward ensuring that you are as healthy as possible as you start your new life as a family.

6

Bringing Baby Home

Charlotte, a patient I began to see soon after the birth of her first child, said to me, "I couldn't believe it when they handed me the baby when it was time to go home. I mean, were they crazy? I didn't know how to take care of a baby. I'd never even changed a diaper before. And breastfeeding? My milk hadn't come in by the time I'd left the hospital, and I had this screaming infant on my hands. I knew he was hungry, but when I called my doctor, his nurse said whatever you do, don't give the baby a bottle; he'll get nipple confusion. Nipple confusion? What in God's name is nipple confusion? But I was so paranoid that I was going to do something wrong that I think I almost starved the poor child to death those first few days. And Richard kept looking at me like I was supposed to know what to do. All I wanted to do was take the baby back to the hospital and tell them they'd made a big mistake letting me take this child home. I have never felt so scared or so alone."

Why It's Called the Fourth Trimester

Remember when you were thin, having sex, staying up late for parties, and watching *Casablanca* on the late show? Then you were pregnant, awkward, tired, swollen, and unable to see your feet — longing for the time when your baby would be born. Now the baby is here, and this means you've taken the first step toward getting your body back. But it also means there is a whole new person in the world who is suddenly the center of the universe. Negotiating all these transitions is not easy for anyone. Even for a woman who has become accustomed to not being in control of her body, it can be difficult to realize that an eight-pound, twenty-inch baby is now in charge.

The first six weeks of having a new baby are some of the most challenging weeks in a woman's life. It's a relief to be done with pregnancy and delivery, but now there is a small stranger who demands continuous attention. The problem is, babies can't tell you what they need. Are they tired, hungry, bored, lonely, or wet? In those first weeks, learning your baby's crying language is a major developmental task for both you and the baby.

Delivering a baby is tremendous physical work — think of it as major surgery (having a C-section literally is) — and yet the American health system sends mother and baby home twenty-four hours after delivery. The combination of hormonal changes and the anxiety of not knowing what the infant needs will take its toll on any new mother's moods. In addition to sleep deprivation and soreness, the demands of learning to breastfeed are significant. This transition, though long awaited, is shocking to mother and baby. That's why the first three months of the baby's life are often called the fourth trimester.

The infant is no longer inside, but mother and child are still tied together. Now, however, their needs are not always in harmony. When the baby needs food, the mother may be in the middle of her own meal. When the baby wakes up from a nap, the mother may just have fallen asleep. The new mother finds herself in the middle of an unpredictable roller coaster ride, which she can't just stop and get off. For a woman used to schedules and order, these first several weeks can feel chaotic. And yet everyone is saying how happy she must be.

As during the first trimester, her body is washed in mood-altering chemicals. Immediately after the placenta is delivered, estrogen levels and progesterone levels plummet, and if the infant is being breastfed, they will take several months to equilibrate. New hormones, oxytocin and prolactin, become prominent in the breastfeeding mother. Just like estrogen and progesterone, these hormones have both positive and negative effects on the new mother's moods.

Despite the excitement and joy of the new arrival, these first six weeks are a trial for everyone. Not much is predictable about this time. For a day or two, the infant may need to eat every two or three hours, then every four or five, and then back to two or three. You thought you'd have a chance to take a nap, but there's a diaper to change, a neighbor brings over a casserole, or your milk lets down and you have to change your shirt. The biggest challenge new mothers face is simply to keep going during this tumultuous time before the newborn matures and a more predictable schedule emerges.

No matter how many books you read, nothing can prepare you for the fact that you are totally responsible for another human being's life.

❦

LISA, A PRACTICING ATTORNEY in a small law firm, came to my office three weeks after the delivery of her first child, a boy.

She and her husband, Ed, had agreed to wait to have a child until Lisa was out of law school and had found a job. She described her marriage and life as being good — until recently. "What brought you in to see me today?" I asked.

Lisa began to cry quietly. "I always knew I wanted children," she said. "I love kids. Ed and I waited a long time to have a child, and I was so excited when we finally got pregnant."

Lisa stopped talking and looked at me with tears running down her face. "And now . . . ?" I gently probed.

"Now . . . Now, I just want someone to take him away. I don't think I want a baby anymore, and I know that's not the way I'm supposed to feel. I look at him and just ask myself what have we done?"

I waited for her sobbing to subside, then said, "You know, it sounds as if you're having a really hard time with all the changes a new baby brings. How is your husband adjusting?"

"He's miserable, too. The last two weekends since we brought the baby home, we've just sat in the house. It just seems so overwhelming to get everything organized to be able to go out. What if I need to breastfeed the baby while we're out? Do I feed him in the middle of the mall or go into the bathroom? What if he starts crying and doesn't stop? When will I ever get to be alone with my husband again?"

Lisa hadn't slowed down during her pregnancy. She'd left work to go straight to the hospital to have the baby. The delivery had been extraordinarily easy. Lisa's large family and friends showered her and her husband with gifts and casseroles, and for the first ten days Lisa barely had a chance to hold the baby. Then everybody went home. Lisa and Ed were alone, and they were terrified. They were now in charge of knowing when the baby was wet, hungry, or tired. They were the only ones that small creature had to rely on for absolutely everything, and they felt totally ignorant. How were they supposed to know why their baby was crying? And if feeding, changing, and rocking didn't work, what then?

I knew that this state of high agitation would resolve itself in a few weeks. I explained to Lisa that it takes a while to establish a rhythm between baby and parents. By six weeks, she and her baby would no longer be strangers but intimate partners. She would instinctively know things about him and be able to read his moods despite the fact that no words passed between them. In the meantime, she needed to turn to friends and family to help. No one expected Lisa and Ed to do it all by themselves in the beginning. And most people love being around newborns. I told Lisa not to expect herself to be an expert on newborns by week two. By week six, however, she *would* be the expert on her baby.

I assured Lisa that she could come back to see me at any time, but if she and Ed could just hold on for a few more weeks, things would get better. She didn't believe me entirely; she and Ed were truly distraught. I asked her to call me the following week to let me know how she was doing. I didn't hear from her for a month, so I called her. Things were fine, and she hadn't thought to call me because the crisis that had brought her to my office had disappeared.

ONCE THAT BABY is placed in your arms, there is no turning back. It doesn't matter who you are or what your experience is; the arrival of a newborn is scary. Before I went to medical school, I worked as a neonatal intensive care nurse. I took care of the tiniest, most critically ill newborns. Even so, I'll never forget the panic I felt one night after having my first child. We had been home from the hospital for about two weeks, and all of the relatives had left to resume their lives. I was changing my daughter's diaper in the middle of the night and noticed that the diaper was full of bright pumpkin-colored stool. I had changed a lot of diapers and had never seen anything quite that color. I woke up my husband and asked him to look.

"You've got to be kidding," he said. "It's the middle of the night. You want me to look at a dirty diaper?"

"It's a funny color. I don't think it's supposed to be that color."

"It looks fine to me. Go back to sleep." He rolled over and did just that.

My mind started swirling. Breastfed babies were supposed to have yellow stools. But this was orange. Could there be something wrong with her liver? Or did she have some awful metabolic disorder? I started to scare myself. At two o'clock in the morning, I got out of bed, turned on the light, and started reading my pediatrics textbooks. I scoured the pages for anything I could find about stool color. Buttery yellow, golden — nothing I read said anything about orange. In tears, I again woke up my husband.

I told him that none of my books said anything about bright orange stools and that something must be terribly wrong. I managed to get him frightened, too, and he suggested that we call the pediatrician. I imagined making that call at what was now three in the morning: "Hello, I'm calling because my baby had orange poop in her diaper." Then I imagined the long silence on the other end of the line. Imagining waking the pediatrician up in the middle of the night and the shame I would feel was enough to calm me down. I turned to my husband and said, "Never mind. It's probably okay." With that, I pushed the books off the bed, turned out the light, and went to sleep. He lay there for another hour worrying. The next morning, everything was fine. Reason always returns when the sun comes up.

Stay in Your Pajamas

Savor the time you have to nurture and learn about your newborn, and to nourish your body and spirit. Not to do so invites fatigue, irritability, and potentially depression. You will never have another chance to snuggle and cuddle with this baby and to pay attention solely to your newborn's and your needs. The first six weeks can be magical if you allow yourself the time to enjoy it. Rushing to do laundry and grocery shopping or returning to work before you and the baby have a chance to establish a rhythm can rob you of the magic.

TINA CAME TO my office when her baby was four weeks old. She was beautifully dressed and made-up. She had an adorable baby girl who looked as if she belonged on the cover of *Parents* magazine. I was jealous that anyone could look so good so soon after delivering a baby. After my pregnancies, it had taken me eighteen months to get back in shape, no matter how hard I tried. I asked her why she had come to see me.

She gave me a tight, perfectly lipsticked smile, and then she crumpled and said, "I'm miserable. This is so much harder than I expected. I can't sleep, and I cry all the time. I have never been like this before. I can run three community events without thinking about it, but this tiny baby has me totally undone."

I wondered how much energy it cost her to keep up appearances. I couldn't imagine how she did it. "You look like you're doing amazingly well," I said. "No one would ever imagine you were struggling so much. Have you told anyone how you're feeling?"

"No. I don't want to seem as if I'm unhappy with my baby. My sister just had a miscarriage a few months ago, and I should feel really grateful that everything turned out so well. I don't want to complain, and I *am* grateful. It's just that . . . I just didn't think it would be so hard. I'm so tired. I can't even manage to get myself dressed until right before my husband comes home. And forget about dinner. I'm lucky if we even have anything in the house to eat. My husband's been really great and hasn't complained, but he works all day, and all I do is stay home. I should at least have dinner ready for him when he gets there. I feel so guilty. I think there's something wrong with me. Everyone else seems able to handle having kids."

This woman was only four weeks postdelivery, and she expected that she should be able to function just as she had before the baby was born. She was doomed if she thought she could take care of her new baby, clean the house, cook a gourmet meal, organize a community event, and not be exhausted and frustrated at the end of the day.

And her comment that all she did was stay home? In some ways, it is much easier going to a busy office and dealing with intelligent adults than it is trying to manage a baby who can't communicate in any way besides crying. There's nothing more stressful or frightening than a baby who won't stop crying. You've fed him, changed him, and rocked him, but still the screaming continues. At moments like that, all you want to do is hand the baby to someone else and leave. But there's no one to hand him to, and you can't go anywhere. It can be emotionally and physically exhausting.

When I asked Tina who had helped her after her daughter was born, she said, "My husband stayed home from work for two days, but we really couldn't afford for him to take much more time off. He owns his own business, and there just isn't anyone who can take over when he's away."

"Did your mother or your husband's mother come at all?"

"My mom came and stayed with me for a week after my husband went back to work. She has five children and showed me how to take care of a baby. I was doing okay while she was here, but the night before she was supposed to get on the plane, I totally panicked. I realized I was going to be left all alone with the baby. Mom had to get back to work. I didn't want to make her feel bad by letting her know how scared I was. This shouldn't be that big a deal."

Tina and her husband had just moved into a new neighborhood. They had not yet met their neighbors or found a church close to home. Most of Tina's friends were from work. She saw some moms in the neighborhood walking together with their strollers, but she didn't know how to meet them.

After the first two weeks, all her help disappeared, and she was on her own. Her husband worked twelve to fourteen hours a day. Even though her world had been turned upside down, she felt as if everyone expected her to go on as usual and do just fine. "After all," she told herself, "women have been having babies for centuries."

She was right. In our culture, independence and self-sufficiency are highly valued, and asking for help signifies weakness or neediness. Rest and taking care of oneself is often seen as laziness and selfishness. But being at home all day with a small child is a risk factor for postpartum depression.

For many women, two weeks is not enough time to feel competent about being alone with a tiny baby. At two weeks, you are still exhausted and getting mostly interrupted sleep. The baby is not on any schedule, and you are still trying to figure out how often he'll want to eat and how many diapers to buy. If you're trying to breastfeed, two weeks is just about the time you might *start* feeling as if you and the baby know what you're doing. For some mothers, breastfeeding is still a mystery after two weeks.

Tina's mother-in-law lived nearby and did not work. Tina said she was available and willing to help but was afraid of intruding and getting in the way. Tina didn't want to ask her mother-in-law for help for fear of inconveniencing her. But she was even more concerned about making her mother-in-law think that she wasn't capable of taking care of a baby.

While Tina was telling me her story, I could see that she was exhibiting some symptoms of depression. She believed that asking for help was not an option. At times like this, I become very firm about what I think is necessary to protect the mother's health. "You need to get some help during the day so that you can take a break," I told her. "If you don't get more rest, I am worried that you may become depressed enough that we will need to start you on medication. I don't want you to get to a place where you feel that bad."

"But there's no one who can help me," she replied. "I can't ask my mother to come back."

"What about your mother-in-law?"

"I don't want her to know how much I'm struggling. I don't want her to know that I had to see a psychiatrist. She'll think I'm such a screwup. She won't want me to be married to her son anymore."

It is extremely common for people not to want anyone to know that they have seen a mental health professional. If you need to see a psychiatrist, it must mean that you're really crazy. That's often a new mother's worst fear — that I will confirm that she is "crazy."

"Well, you don't have to tell her you've seen a psychiatrist; that's up to you," I said. "But you could tell her that you've been having a harder time than you thought you would and that you could really use her help. Tell her your obstetrician said you need more rest. If she could come over for four or five hours in the middle of the day for a few days, so that you could take a nap, it might make a huge difference.

"I think you've expected too much of yourself too soon. You just had a baby four weeks ago. You need to put your pajamas on and get back into bed."

"What do you mean?" Tina asked.

"You have just had a baby. It is too soon to be up and running around. You should still be in bed in your pajamas breastfeeding your baby and sleeping. I want you to get back in bed for a week and not do anything but be a new mom. You shouldn't be worried about picking up the house or cooking dinner. No one cares what your house looks like. Everyone realizes you've just had a baby. Maybe some of your friends could bring meals for a few days."

"I don't know. I don't know if I can ask people to do that."

"You really don't have a choice."

Tina confided to her mother-in-law that she was having a hard time and asked her to help. Much to Tina's surprise, her mother-in-law really pitched in. Although Tina didn't get back in bed, she quit trying to be a superwoman and took things more slowly. Her friends wanted to be supportive, and she ended up with a freezer full of casseroles, enough for the next several weeks. With sleep and a slower pace, things improved greatly. By the time the baby was eight weeks old, Tina felt like her old, on-top-of-things self.

What About Breastfeeding?

We all know the virtues of breastfeeding. Mother's milk is perfectly designed by nature to nourish the baby. It is amazing how the mother's body adapts to what her baby needs. If an infant is born prematurely, the milk the mother makes is uniquely suited for that infant. As the baby grows, the composition of proteins and fats in the milk changes to meet the infant's changing needs.

Not only is breast milk nutritionally sound, but it also offers many other advantages for a baby. A breastfed baby has fewer ear infections, less colic, fewer gastrointestinal problems, and fewer allergies, and he or she can fight infections better. In light of this abundance of positive effects, the American Academy of Pediatrics recommends that all infants be breastfed. Currently, the recommendation is to nurse until the infant is one year of age, if possible.

We know the advantages for the mother as well. Women who breastfeed their infants have a decreased risk for breast cancer. They may find it easier to lose weight after delivery. There is also a great emotional component to breastfeeding for both mother and baby. Mothers will often talk of the blissful experience of holding their babies in their arms, skin to skin, and knowing that they are providing everything the babies need to grow. The hormone oxytocin, which accompanies breastfeeding, enhances feelings of love and encourages the mother to nurture and bond with her infant.

Breastfeeding is wonderful — unless it isn't. Some women don't want to breastfeed. For whatever reason, they don't like the idea of it. Some women are modest, and the thought of being so exposed is uncomfortable. Some worry that they may find breastfeeding sexually arousing. And some women are concerned that they won't be successful at it: their breasts are too small or their nipples are inverted.

Often physical, not psychological, discomfort is the problem. No one warns you about this, but in the beginning it *hurts* to breastfeed. Your nipples can become extremely tender and sore.

When the baby latches on to the breast to nurse, the pain can be severe. A tiny infant can create incredible suction when nursing. It is not uncommon for a woman's nipples to bleed in the beginning if she nurses too frequently or if the infant is a particularly vigorous feeder. Breastfeeding is something that mother and baby have to learn together. It can take several days to several weeks for both to become comfortable with nursing.

It's frustrating to try to calm a crying baby, and a woman may end up nursing for hours on end in an attempt to get the baby to quiet down. New mothers often assume that every time the baby cries, he's hungry. Sometimes they feel as if they have their shirts off for most of the day. In addition, unless you weigh the baby before and after every feeding, it's impossible to know how much a breastfed baby has eaten. This can cause great anxiety about whether the baby has gotten enough milk.

And then there is the issue of loss. Although breastfeeding is in many ways a wonderful thing, it means the mother gives up all sense of personal space. When your baby is hungry and ready to eat, for the most part it's your job to unbutton your shirt and provide the food. This could be in the middle of the mall, at church, or on an airplane. There aren't many places designed to accommodate a breastfeeding mother and child. I have nursed a child while sitting on a toilet in a bathroom stall, one of the most common spots to find some breastfeeding privacy.

A breastfeeding mother is tied to her child in a way that no one else is. Unless she is able to pump milk for a bottle, she is the only one who can feed her baby. If everyone is sitting around enjoying a holiday dinner and the baby cries, Mom is the one whose dinner gets cold. Unless she's willing to nurse at the table, she winds up alone in the next room listening to everyone tell stories and laugh while she waits for the baby to finish nursing. In the middle of the night, there is no trading off the feeding.

Dad can get the baby ready for nursing, but Mom has to do the actual work.

Sometimes this is hard to tolerate. I was good for about six months. After that, I was tired of being tied down to a breast-feeding baby. I wanted my body back.

Women have been taught that breastfeeding is the best option for new babies. Some physicians tell their patients quite adamantly that breastfeeding is the only option, and for as long as is humanly possible. Lactation nurses and breastfeeding support groups focus on helping women have a positive breastfeeding experience. All that is great, but some mothers can't, or shouldn't, breastfeed, and the guilt associated with being an unsuccessful breastfeeder can be enormous. Some women have a terrible time giving themselves permission to stop, even when it's not working.

❧

CORINNE WAS LOOKING forward to the birth of her baby and made sure everything was ready for him. She couldn't wait to hold her son in her arms. The baby was going to be called Thomas, after Corinne's father, who died when she was a girl.

Her water broke in the middle of the night, and seven hours later Thomas was born without complications. Both sides of the family were in attendance, and the nurses finally had to kick everyone out of the room so that the new parents could try to get some sleep.

"It all seemed so perfect," Corinne told me six weeks later. "It was just as I'd imagined. I even got through it without any pain medication. He was so beautiful, and I felt so happy. And then we went home, and I don't know what happened."

Corinne was sitting in my office. Her husband, John, and baby Thomas were waiting for her in the waiting room. John had called Corinne's doctor and told him that she was crying all the time. The obstetrician had called me and asked if I could see her as soon as possible. He was worried that she was seriously depressed and might need medication.

"Tell me what happened after you got home," I said to Corinne. "When did you start feeling bad?"

"You know, it's hard to sort out. It seems like things never got on track. Thomas doesn't breastfeed very well, and I'm not sure I have enough milk. He just keeps screaming and screaming. It's awful. He wants to nurse all the time. It seems as if all I do is sit around with my shirt off."

"Are you still nursing, or have you stopped?"

"I'm still trying, but it's not going very well. Thomas cries all the time and doesn't seem to want to latch on to the breast. He'll suck for a few seconds and then start screaming." Corinne looked as if she was at her limit and any more stress would topple her. I asked what I thought was an obvious question — "Why not stop?" — and she started to sob. "I can't stop breastfeeding. My sister breastfed her baby until she was two and keeps telling me it will get better. My pediatrician says that breast milk is the best thing for the baby. He wants me to nurse until the baby's at least one year old."

I tried to give her some reasonable advice. "Breastfeeding is best for a baby, but not if it's making both you and him miserable. Are you making enough milk?"

"I think so. I've been pumping after I nurse the baby so that I'll have something to feed him between feedings. I'm getting about two ounces every time I pump."

"How often are you nursing and pumping?"

"I've lost track. The baby cries all the time. I try to pump at least every three hours so that I can have some milk stored, and then in between the pumping, I'm trying to feed him. I didn't think it was supposed to be this hard."

"Do you have any help, or are you trying to do this all on your own?"

"My mother stayed with us for two weeks, and I sobbed when she left. I couldn't believe she was going to leave me all alone. I was so scared, and John had to go back to work. I started to really lose it then. The baby cries all the time, and I'm in the house by myself. I can't even shower or get dressed. John comes home from work and asks what I've done all day, and I just start crying. I practically throw the baby at him and get in bed. All I can do is pull the covers up over my head and cry. I'm so scared I'm doing something to hurt the baby."

Corinne was sobbing. Her face was puffy, and she had dark circles under her eyes. I didn't think she'd washed her hair in several days. "Corinne, you're exhausted, and you're becoming depressed," I said. "It isn't supposed to be this hard. It isn't your fault, and you're not a terrible mother. You need some help. I have to ask you some hard questions. Are you having any thoughts at all of hurting yourself or the baby?"

"No, no, no. I don't want to hurt him or myself. I just want to go away and never come back."

I was worried that Corinne might be suffering from a depression severe enough that she would need medication. But I also wondered whether if she stopped nursing and was able to get more sleep, her stress might decrease, and she might start feeling better.

"Corinne, we need to talk about changing your stress level and getting you more sleep. If things keep going the way they are, you could become depressed enough to need medication. If you can get some uninterrupted sleep and take away the stress you are experiencing with breastfeeding, things may get a lot better. Is there anyone who can come to stay with you and help with the baby?"

"My mom just went home; she has to work. I can't ask her to come back."

"How about a sister or your mother-in-law? Anybody who can come and help you for at least a week, until you start feeling better."

"There's nobody like that. My sisters are coming in a couple of weeks, but I'll be alone until then."

"I don't think being alone is such a good idea. We have to think of someone who can help. Could your sisters come earlier?"

It is hard to ask for help, but help is exactly what Corinne needed. Depression makes it almost impossible to take care of yourself, let alone a new baby. And the anxiety brought on by a baby who's having difficulty breastfeeding can get the best of even the most experienced mother.

"The fact that you're feeling bad is not your fault," I said. "You haven't done anything wrong, and the way you feel doesn't mean that you are a bad mother. You don't want to feel this way, and this is not at all what you expected. I think the worst part is that you had looked forward to bringing your new baby home and enjoying him. And now you are miserable. And no matter how hard you try, you can't talk yourself out of it or fix it on your own. You need help, and we may need to talk about a medication to treat your depression."

"I don't want to take anything," Corinne said. "That would really make me feel like a failure. I'll be okay."

"I think we can wait on that to see how you do in the next few days. But you've got to get your family to help you, and you have to get some sleep. For the next several nights, somebody else needs to get up with the baby. Six hours of uninterrupted sleep for a few nights, and you will most likely start to feel better."

"But what about breastfeeding?"

It is my job to help people decide what is best for them. Sometimes I need to give them permission to make a difficult decision that is in their best interest.

"I think you need to stop breastfeeding," I said. "It's not working for you or the baby and is adding way too much stress to your life. It's okay not to breastfeed. The differences between breast milk and formula aren't enough to justify your being so miserable. There may be some people who disagree, but you have to do what is right for you. You are the only one who truly knows how difficult these last four weeks have been."

I saw her face start to soften and show relief. "You also need some help. The best thing you can do right now is to give yourself a break. It's going to take you a few weeks to get back on your feet, and you need some support."

"I guess I could ask my mom to come back. Maybe we can send her the money for a plane ticket."

"If you told her what was going on, she'd come right back. Why don't you have your husband come in, and we'll talk over these plans with him."

For Corinne, stopping the breastfeeding was the right decision. It was better for both her and the baby. More than mother's milk, a baby needs a mom who is calm, not stressed and not depressed. Infants pick up on a mother's tension. Not only does stress decrease a woman's milk supply, but a baby also responds poorly to the mother's anxiety and becomes difficult to soothe.

After only a week of improved sleep and a baby who was feeding well with a bottle, Corinne felt like she was getting back to her old self. She began to enjoy being a mother. Even though she was disappointed that breastfeeding hadn't worked out, she was relieved that she felt much more in control. At her final appointment, Corinne said to me, "This really was the right decision for us. Maybe next time, breastfeeding will be an option. But for now, I feel good about my choice."

Nurturing Yourself

TAKE CARE OF YOURSELF FIRST should be at the top of every instruction sheet given to new mothers. The demands are overwhelming in those first few weeks. Managing your infant, dealing with helpful (or intrusive) family, and trying to negotiate new roles with your husband are all gigantic tasks. But you do come first in an important way: you need to be strong and reasonably stable for the baby. It's important to let as many things go as possible so that you can concentrate on both yourself and the baby.

Take weight, for example. One of the first things many new mothers worry about is losing their pregnancy weight. It should be the last thing. Many women gain between twenty and forty pounds during pregnancy, and it doesn't all miraculously disappear when the baby is born. If you are breastfeeding, your body will protect its fat stores to make sure there is always enough nutrition available for your baby. Although breastfeeding over many months may be an excellent way to lose your pregnancy weight gradually, an extra five to ten pounds may linger until you have finished nursing.

Many women struggle to lose the weight they gained during pregnancy. Even so, immediately postpartum is not the time to fret about weight loss. Your body needs to adjust to not being pregnant any longer. It takes many weeks for your uterus to return to its pre-pregnancy size. It takes months for your abdominal muscles to tighten up and your skin to regain its elasticity. In all actuality, your body will never totally be the same again.

After having four children, my friend Joanne looks exactly as she did in high school. When she left the hospital after having each of her children, she could not only wear her blue jeans but also zip them up. She is an anomaly. A few women in the world are fortunate enough to have miracle bodies. Do not compare yourself to them; most of us can't rebound nearly that fast. And it's not because of laziness. Losing weight postpartum takes time and work. Give yourself a break; do not try to diet immediately after giving birth. If you are breastfeeding, you need to make sure you are getting enough calories to sustain your milk supply and nourish your baby.

It's great if you have friends and family to provide meals those first few weeks at home. It's important that you eat nutritious, well-balanced meals and drink plenty of fluids. Keep a cooler filled with water and juice by your bed. Every time you breastfeed, replenish your own body with plenty of fluids. Having fresh fruit nearby is also a good idea. Easily accessible nutrition is an important part of the healing process. It also encourages you to stay in bed and let others take care of you.

❧

I'M GOING TO repeat myself: the person most often overlooked when bringing a new baby home is the mother. No matter how many children you've had or how much experience, being exhausted and anxious is part and parcel of the first weeks of motherhood. That's because every baby is different. Some sleep well; some are awake all the time. Some are peaceful; some startle at the slightest noise. If the baby is a good sleeper, the mother worries that she may be sick or even dying. If the baby has trouble nursing, the mother worries that he is starving. The slightest cry has parents jumping out of their seats, and long periods of fussiness are enough to make any parent want to leave and never come back. That anxious period is short-lived, as mother and child begin to understand each other's signals, but the exhaustion goes on for a very long time.

Sleep can be the most difficult thing for a new mother to achieve and may be the most important. Without adequate sleep, the mother is irritable, tearful, confused, and at greater risk for depression. Every pregnant woman needs to plan for adequate sleep in the immediate postpartum period. It may take some creativity to find time to sleep, and it will definitely take the cooperation of others. The baby has a schedule of his own, and you can't depend on him to know that you're so tired you can barely function. Nannies, friends, and family members need to pitch in. Getting several hours of deep sleep in a row may be one of the best ways to ensure that both mom and baby stay healthy and thrive.

Taking care of yourself physically, emotionally, and spiritually is a way to ensure that you will be able to take care of others. As a psychiatrist, I spend my days engaged with patients in an intensely emotional way. I give them support, understanding, and empathy. I sit with them while they work through painful experiences. All of this is done without asking them to provide me with the same support in return. It can be exhausting and wrenching to be so available to others. To do my work well, I must feel fulfilled and centered in my own life. I have to make sure I work reasonable hours, have stable personal relationships, and take enough breaks away from work to recharge my battery.

These same principles can be applied to parenting. A valued colleague of mine, Sherri Duson, is a marriage and family therapist who works with women, couples, and families as they nego-

tiate the rough terrain of parenthood. She has developed a c
list for new mothers to help remind them to pay attention to
their own needs. I think it's a wonderful reminder of what
women need to do, every day, to stay healthy.

THE WELL MOM CHECKLIST

- ☐ 1. Have I eaten enough nutritious food today?
- ☐ 2. Have I slept at least five hours or taken a nap?
- ☐ 3. Have I bathed or showered today?
- ☐ 4. Have I exercised at least ten minutes today?
- ☐ 5. Have I had at least ten minutes of quiet time for reflection and renewal today?
- ☐ 6. Have I let myself laugh today?
- ☐ 7. Have I let others help me today?
- ☐ 8. Have I kissed my baby and told him or her "I love you" today?
- ☐ 9. Have I talked to at least one adult today about how I'm (not the baby is) doing?
- ☐ 10. Have I forgiven myself for my mistakes today?

© 2000 by Sherry J. Duson, M.A.

It is hard to get through the first six weeks with a new baby.
Even if you've been through it before, you are likely to forget
just how hard it is. This period really is a gateway to the rest of
your life. Things almost invariably get better. The rashes subside, the schedule smoothes out, husband and wife get in the
swing of parenthood, and that most adorable creature on the
planet begins to gurgle and smile. It seems to me that if you can
get through the first six weeks with a new baby, everything else
(for a while) is easier.

That's good, because being a mother is a full-time, lifelong
job. How you mother will have enduring effects on your child.

That can be an overwhelming responsibility. Fortunately, children are resilient and can absorb a lot of mistakes with no ill effects. Sometimes being able to laugh at yourself is the most important skill you can have. It is okay not to get it right all the time. It is okay sometimes to want to run away. It is okay sometimes to want to hold your child for hours because she is so precious. It is okay.

· TIPS ·

The first six weeks are all about rest and recovery for both you and your baby. Your job is to feed yourself and your newborn and to allow both of you to get to know each other's rhythms. The key words are "rest" and "more rest." Enjoy this special time when you can shut out the world and get to know your new family member.

1. *Visitors.* If you thought you couldn't sleep in the hospital, wait until you get home. The doorbell and phone may never stop ringing. Just when you think you've settled your newborn down and you have time to take a nap, Aunt Millie knocks on the door. Even if you have a cute sign on the door such as SHH, BABY SLEEPING, Aunt Millie is sure that you don't mean *her*. Appoint a sentry — someone to turn away visitors who show up unannounced. Don't even let them in the door. Or post a sign saying, "We're so sorry; we're all unavailable at the moment. We'll be receiving visitors tomorrow between one and two. Hope you'll stop by then."

You get to decide when you are ready to have people come by. Limit the time you are willing to be disturbed. Pick an afternoon or an evening when you feel up to having one or two visitors. This is your time to take care of yourself, not to make everyone in the neighborhood happy. If they truly care about you, they will realize that having a new baby at home is hard work, and you're not being rude, just protective.

A friend of mine turned off the ringer on her phone and had the following message on her machine: "Thank you for calling about the new baby. Mother and baby are doing well and are either resting or feeding. Please leave a message, and we'll call you back when we can. We appreciate all of your good wishes. We're having a ball." This simple message left her long stretches of quiet time. Her husband would check the messages at the end of the day and return phone calls at a convenient time.

2. *A bedside cooler.* Your main job is to stay in bed and nourish yourself and your baby. Imagine making a nest where you can be comfortable and have easy access to everything you need. Place a cooler full of water, juice, fruit, and other nourishing foods beside your bed or sofa. If you are breastfeeding, it is important that you remain well hydrated and take in healthy calories. A cooler makes it easy for you to reach down and grab something to drink when you are thirsty. It is much harder to stay well hydrated if you have to ask someone to bring you something.

3. *Diapers close at hand.* You have a lovely nursery for your baby, with adorable curtains and bedding. The only trouble is that you have to leave your room to get there. The baby monitor is fine for when the baby is sleeping, but it doesn't help when you need to change a diaper. And early on, you are changing diapers every hour or so. So make it easy on yourself; have a supply of diapers, sleepers, and a diaper pail in the same room where you have set yourself up to rest. Don't make recovery harder than it already is. Who cares if you use the brand-new diaper pail in the beautiful nursery or temporarily use a trash bag in the corner of your room? Not as pretty, but so much more convenient.

4. *Sleeping arrangements.* For the first six weeks, it is easier to have the baby beside your bed in a bassinet than down the hall in the nursery. How much easier it is to reach beside you to pick up the baby to nurse than to go down the hall every hour. It's also easier to check on all those gurgles and whimpers that you're learning to understand. At three in the morning, it's a long walk to the nursery, and sounds on a baby monitor may be a lot more frightening than when they are happening right beside you.

There is an exception to this advice. If you are unable to sleep through the little noises a newborn makes, you may need to put the bassinet on the other side of the room or next to your partner's side of the bed. If that doesn't work, it may help for you to sleep in another room and let your husband bring you the baby when it's time to nurse. Adequate sleep for Mom is crucial during this early stage, and you may have to get creative to make sure you get enough.

Many couples work out a schedule where both get sleep and both help with feedings. If you are breastfeeding, have your partner bring the baby to you, then change her diaper and put her back to sleep when you are finished nursing. This will make it easier for you to fall back asleep after nursing.

If you are bottle-feeding, you can alternate feedings. Or you can take the two o'clock shift while he takes the five or six o'clock shift before he goes to work. It's possible to work out an arrangement where both of you are getting at least four hours of uninterrupted sleep. It's not just Mom who's tired when a new baby is brought home, and Dad is not the only one working. Both of you need to participate in the care of your newborn, and both of you need rest.

5. *Forget fashion.* Wear comfortable clothes during the first six weeks at home. Don't even try to fit into your old clothes; it will only make you feel bad. You're not supposed to fit into

them; you just had a baby! It's okay to wear your husband's sweatpants, but why not have some of your own that don't make you feel so ungainly? Remember, you are not dressing for work or to go out to lunch with your friends. You are dressing for comfort and ease.

6. *Sibling survival.* It's difficult to bring a new baby home to other children. No matter how old they are, they will have to adjust to the intruder. An older child will naturally fear that Mommy and Daddy will no longer have time for him or that the baby is now his parents' favorite. And it's not just other children who may be jealous; mothers and fathers also may miss that special time they shared with an older child. Everyone will eventually get adjusted, but there are ways to make sure these normal jealous feelings are resolved quickly and easily.

In the first few days and weeks at home, when there is more help in the house, set aside some special time for each child. Grandparents can be wonderful at entertaining other children. Perhaps Grandma can take each child out for an hour or two so that no one else is competing for her attention. Most important, use other adults to watch the baby for at least half an hour each day so that you can give each older sibling your undivided attention. (This doesn't mean reading the older child a story while you are breastfeeding. This means reading a story and cuddling in your bed while the baby is in another room.) Tell the child that this is his time to spend just with you. Dads should have some special time with other children, too. Although this won't resolve jealous feelings, it will help calm unspoken fears of being cast aside.

Many families have told me during the first several weeks that they are amazed at how well their other children are adjusting to the new baby. The older children are covering the newborn with kisses, wanting to hold her, and even trying to help feed her and change her diaper. This is great, but in my experience, sibling rivalry starts in earnest around six weeks. This is when parents may notice more temper tantrums and regressed behavior in older children. The novelty of the newborn wears off, and older siblings realize that she is there to stay. Don't worry; this behavior won't last, and giving siblings special time will go a long way toward settling things down.

7

The New Normal

It was a trend for a time to have BABY ON BOARD signs in the windows of cars carrying children. The message was a mixture of pride in the precious cargo being carried and a stern warning to be cautious when driving near this car. During the first six weeks of a newborn's life, your baby may seem like a wriggling alien, demanding nothing but food and comfort. But by the seventh or eighth week, a personality has begun to emerge. There *is* a baby on board!

The chaos of those first few weeks eases as you and your baby become more comfortable with each other and a routine starts to develop. The baby's schedule still demands flexibility, but changes occur every few weeks as opposed to hour by hour. As much as it may feel as if life is slowly regaining some sense of normalcy, however, in some ways this is when the real work of parenting begins. All the extra help has gone home, and the hoopla has died down, but the baby is here to stay. You begin to realize that you've signed on for a lifetime commitment and there is no going back. I describe the process during this six-week period as finding the new normal.

The new normal constantly changes. There's an adjustment when your baby starts to roll over and you can no longer leave him in the middle of the bed surrounded by pillows. Then he crawls and walks and wants to go on dates and drive the family car. Fortunately, by the time all of those things happen, you will have a little more experience under your belt. For now, you're beginning to realize that life as you knew it has changed forever — mostly for the better, but also with some difficult challenges to face.

There are four major areas in which profound adjustments take place. First, women must reexamine their definitions of a good mother. Second, parents must face and deal with their ambivalence about having children now that the baby is here. Third, couples need to find the new normal of intimacy and sexuality. And fourth, many women must confront the challenge of going back to work, which generally happens toward the end of this period.

The Good Enough Mother

A fear lurks inside most women that maybe they aren't good mothers. Being in charge of another human being is an enormous responsibility. What if you're not up to the job? Will you fail your baby if you give her the wrong food or let her cry too long? What if you feel like abandoning your baby, or worse? I've not yet spoken to a mother who hasn't confessed that at some point, she understood how a parent could shake his or her baby when nothing would stop the infant from crying. The difference between "us" and "them" is that we walk out of the room before something bad happens. Having the thought doesn't make you a bad mother. Caring for a child is a difficult job, and there is so much pressure to get it right — all the time, every time, and with no room for mistakes.

Is it possible for anyone to live up to the standards women set for themselves? When you're frustrated, annoyed with your child, can't imagine ever liking him again, or want to take him back to where he came from, as long as that is nowhere near where you are — does that make you a bad mother? Are mothers allowed to say these things out loud, or do they have to keep these thoughts to themselves? Are you thinking there's something wrong with me to talk like this, or are you too familiar with those feelings? Motherhood isn't like reality TV — you can't turn it off and wait a week for the next episode. It takes constant hard work and attention, and it's not always fun. Sometimes it's not even mostly fun.

There is no such thing as a perfect mother. I love the ideas of the pediatrician and child psychoanalyst D. W. Winnicott, who said that a child needs a "good enough mother" — one who, most of the time, is loving and attentive and puts the child's needs above her own. That doesn't mean that she is that way all the time. Sometimes she is angry, irrational, and totally selfish. Sometimes she feels as if she hates her child and can't wait to get away from him. But the important thing is that more often than not, she does a pretty good job, sometimes even a great one.

Of course, there are really bad mothers. We hear about them all the time on the news. They are the ones who abuse their children physically, emotionally, and even sexually. They leave their children alone while they go to a bar or out with their boyfriends. If the children of these women survive, they are likely to be severely emotionally disabled and may have to work harder to be good enough parents to their own children. Without help, they may continue the cycle of abuse. It is not hard to identify a truly bad mother.

Fortunately, good enough is good enough. There have been many times when I have been less than a perfect mother. You'd think that a psychiatrist would know better, but psychiatrists are also human beings, at times very flawed human beings. I've had many terrible moments with my children, some of which are truly memorable.

AFTER MY FIRST child, Katie, was born, I was determined to do everything exactly right. There wasn't a child in better hands than mine. As part of my perfect plan, I was going to use cloth diapers. I was sure that they were superior to the disposable kind. They were more "natural," less costly, and friendlier to the environment. I was willing to put up with the smell and the occasional clogged toilet when I accidentally lost my grip while rinsing one.

Cloth diapers required the use of diaper pins. My mother had taught me a trick to ensure that the pins were always sharp and would slide easily through the folded cotton. I had all my diaper pins stuck in a bar of Ivory soap.

Then one day when I was pinning Katie's diaper closed, she began to scream. I was frantic. What was the matter? I picked her up and tried to comfort her, but she was inconsolable. I put her down and checked her diaper. What was wrong? Then I noticed one of the pins going into her thigh and coming out the other side. I had pinned my baby to the diaper! I was panicking as I unclasped the pin and slid it out of her leg. Katie stopped screaming immediately, but my hands were shaking. I wondered what horrible things might happen to her as a result of my mistake. I couldn't think of anything specific, but I was sure that no one had ever done anything so terrible to her baby. My hands shook for the rest of the day, and for a long time I was afraid to tell anyone what I had done. I couldn't imagine how anyone who could pin a diaper to her daughter's leg could be allowed to be a mother.

Katie truly is lucky to have survived a very young woman's first attempts at motherhood. She is also the child whose head I accidentally rolled up in the car's automatic window. When I parked the car in front of our house, I turned around to get her out of her car seat, and realized that her head was out the window and the window was up against her neck. I quickly turned the car back on to get the window down. Katie was fine, but I spent the whole day watching her and making sure she didn't have trouble breathing.

Our family laughs about these two incidents now, but I can still feel the heart-stopping fear and shame I felt then. I've also done my share of screaming, crying, and spanking (even though I don't believe in spanking). The point is that we all have days when we are not at our best, and our children often bear the brunt of it. And contrary to what you might think, there is no one out there who does it much better than you do. You are not the worst mother on your block, in your church, or among your child's friends. You are simply one of the legion of good enough moms.

Ambivalence

All women feel ambivalent about being a mother. It is an enormous sacrifice to raise a child. As I write this, I hear the critic in my head saying, "People reading this are going to think you're a bad person. Children are a privilege and God's gift. What about the women who are desperate to have babies but can't? You shouldn't complain." This is exactly what I mean. Sometimes I am ashamed of my own mixed feelings about motherhood, and I know better.

A colleague of mine, Elizabeth Wallace, wrote a paper titled "Ambivalent Mothers: The Very Last Taboo." She tells about a woman who made the mistake of uttering out loud in a group of mothers, "It's a good thing Jason is in a full-day program, or I'd kill him!" The room grew deathly silent until she said, "Well, you know, I don't mean I'd *really* kill him." Everyone laughed and went back to what they were doing. But when women start to talk like this, it makes people nervous. That woman made the mistake of saying something out loud that all mothers have felt but have kept secret, even from themselves.

Even the woman who lives next door to you — the one who sews all of the costumes for the school play — has moments when she loses it. Some of the women in my office look as if they have it all together. Their children are perfectly dressed, they are room mothers and Scout leaders, and their highlighted hair never shows its roots. They manage to take pictures at all the appropriate times and even remember to get them developed. But sometimes they also wish they were free of the responsibilities of being a mom and wonder what it would be like if they had never had children.

A new mother once asked me whether it was normal to want to get in her car and drive away, leaving her newborn behind. My answer was, "Sometimes." It is not normal to feel that way all of the time. Feeling a total lack of interest in your newborn is one of the symptoms of postpartum depression. But it is normal to feel that way sometimes. It does not make you a bad mother; it just makes you a human being. All mothers struggle with negative feelings about their children. Acknowledging those feelings and not being afraid of them can be the first step in successfully negotiating the transition to motherhood.

❧

ROSA WAS WONDERFULLY honest about the conflicting feelings that many women have after the birth of a baby, particularly their first. A dedicated public school teacher who is "magic" with her six-year-olds, Rosa loves nurturing her darling first graders. You should see the amazing art on the walls of her classroom. Her husband, Mark, is also creative and warm, and they have a strong marriage. Before the birth of their child, Rosa imagined that having her own child would make life even better.

Rosa was raised and educated in Mexico, then came to the United States to study art. After she met Mark and they married, she became a U.S. citizen. She was proud of her accomplishments. Although her family in Mexico had been very poor — her father had worked at a produce stand, and her mother had stayed home with their seven children — Rosa had only good memories of the love and attention her parents had given her.

Rosa's pregnancy hardly interfered with her life. She worked up to the day she delivered a healthy baby girl and had little physical discomfort. Her family came from Mexico for the delivery, and her mother was going to stay on for several months, as Rosa planned to return to work when the baby was six weeks old. She left the hospital anticipating this new, blissful stage of her life.

"I was doing great for the first several weeks," she told me. "I had the normal worries of a new mom, but I don't think it was out of the ordinary. I've been reading on the Internet about baby blues. I think I had that. I cried at the drop of a hat for the first two weeks, but then I was fine. I worried a little bit about having a new baby; I didn't really know what I was doing. My mom had to help me a lot."

Rosa was confused about why she was feeling so uncertain about being a mother. "When did you start doubting yourself?" I asked.

"I don't know. I was doing okay until the baby was about eight weeks old, and then I started to get really anxious. I had been back to work for about two weeks, and I started to get worried about her future."

"What do you mean?"

"I just kept thinking about whether I'd be a good enough mom. I didn't realize how hard it was going to be and how much responsibility having a baby was. They are so small and so incapable of doing anything for themselves. I thought we'd just incorporate her into our lives and keep doing the things we've always done. But I'm so tired all the time. I can't stand listening to my husband talk about his work anymore. I just don't have anything left to give him."

Rosa was feeling overwhelmed by motherhood. She had been totally unprepared for the profound effect that having a baby would have on her husband's and her life. I wondered whether she was struggling with going back to work and whether she felt guilty about leaving her baby to teach other people's children. Maybe she needed permission to stay home with her baby.

"Do you need to work, or is staying home a possibility?" I asked.

Rosa looked at me and was quiet. She said tentatively, "I like to work. After a few weeks at home, I realized I couldn't do that for very much longer. I need adult interaction. I tried to get out to the grocery store and stuff, but that only lasted for a little while." Through tears, she continued, "I don't think I love my baby enough. There's something wrong with me."

I didn't understand. "What do you mean you don't love your baby enough? What do you think is missing?"

"Maybe I'm not cut out to be a mom. Maybe I'm not capable of loving my own child enough. What am I going to do when it's time to teach her the things I teach my kids at school? It's too much. I don't think I can do this."

"Do you mean you feel guilty because you like teaching and aren't devastated by having to leave your baby with your mother?"

"Yes. I think there's something wrong with me."

※

IMAGINING MOTHERHOOD IS very different from experiencing it. It is hard to anticipate all the feelings you will have. Society would have you believe that when you become a mother, a switch turns on in your brain, and you will immediately desire to give up your own life for that of your child. If you prefer to work, our culture implies, you don't love your child enough and aren't a good mother. Women are made to feel that they must sacrifice all of their needs and desires to earn the title "good mother."

Over time, Rosa discovered that being a first-grade teacher and having a baby at home was a fantastic combination. She was exhausted every day, but she found that taking care of her baby helped her to empathize with her kids at school. And during the summer, she could be with the baby all the time and also have a chance to paint and sculpt, which were her great loves. Teaching provided the flexibility Rosa wanted. She was able to create a life that was fulfilling both at work and at home. Rosa was pleased with how things worked out for her. She was both smart and lucky — something we would all like to be.

In our society, there is an underlying attitude that it's acceptable if a mother has to work for financial reasons, but not acceptable if she chooses to work because it is an important part of who she is. The fact that Rosa enjoyed her work and did not feel overwhelming anguish at leaving her baby made her feel extraordinarily guilty. She thought that because she wanted to work, she didn't love her daughter enough.

※

I REMEMBER ONE particular Sunday when my children were younger. That day was a typical day at our house with four children. All of them needed something at exactly the same time, and none of them wanted to wait. One of the boys was being particularly tiresome, having broken the toilet by accidentally flushing a toy Superman down it. The toilet flooded over and I spent two hours snaking the Superman out. Just looking at my son was making my blood boil.

Fortunately, that afternoon he was getting on a plane to Dallas to visit his aunt. All of the children were getting an opportunity to spend some alone time with their favorite aunt. This was a big trip for my son, as he would be making the one-hour flight by himself as an unaccompanied minor. I couldn't wait to get rid of him.

On the way to the airport, he talked incessantly, spilled a drink all over himself, and bumped my arm, causing me to spill hot coffee in my lap. Fortunately we made it to the airport in one piece, negotiated our way through security relatively quickly, and he endeared himself to the elderly woman waiting with him in the preboard area. Once he was allowed to board the airplane, he only ran back down the ramp three times: once to get the backpack he had forgotten, once to ask where his Game Boy was, and the last time to kiss me goodbye.

My heart softened as the other people waiting to board smiled at my beautiful little boy as he wrapped his arms around my waist and gave me a huge hug. "I love you, Mom," he said. "I'll see you in a couple of days." I watched the plane taxi away from the gate and felt mixed emotions. I had never been so ready to send a child off to visit a relative, and yet I missed him already. *That* is ambivalence.

There are many days when I both wish my children hadn't been born and can't imagine my life without them. Some days I actually feel hatred toward them and can't believe that I have been saddled with this burden. Yet at the same time I know that I love my children desperately and would be devastated if anything happened to them.

For some women, the fear of acknowledging any negative feelings about their children causes them to go overboard in the opposite direction. These women never leave their children with a babysitter, are there to meet their children's every need, and never put their own desires first. When this happens, the woman, her partner, and their children suffer. Nobody wins.

The world is not always a nice place. People can be mean, selfish, and even dangerous. No child is the center of the universe and will get everything he or she wants. None of us has someone available twenty-four hours a day to make sure nothing or no one gets in our way. If a child is raised to believe that Mommy will always be there to make things better, he or she is in for big disappointments in life.

Your Relationship with Your Partner

Even when things begin to look up after the first six difficult weeks, the routine of caring for a baby wears a woman down. It can be months until the baby sleeps through the night. Sleep deprivation is a major cause of misery and even depression among new mothers.

That's when the father can play a pivotal role in the mother's well-being. He is the main source of support during pregnancy, labor, and delivery. He is often the only one who is with the mother from beginning to end. After delivery, he can be a buffer between the new mother and the numerous relatives and friends who mean well but may interfere with her rest and privacy.

And yet he is expected to return to work shortly after the birth. Things would be very different if fathers were given the opportunity to continue to play a major role in their babies' earliest weeks. In other industrialized countries, particularly the Netherlands, men are given an equal opportunity to stay home and parent. In the United States, it is still very rare for a man to be given paternity leave as a matter of course. If he wants to spend time with his partner and new baby, he must take vacation time or unpaid leave. Being with a newborn is not a vacation. It is a precious time, but it is hard work.

The mother often buys into the notion that once the father returns to work, he no longer bears any responsibility for the infant's care. She believes that Dad needs to be protected from the exhaustion and stress that come with having a new baby. Some fathers (and mothers) think that staying at home and caring for a baby isn't really work. So when they get home and Mom shoves the baby at them and says, "I just can't take another minute of this child," they feel resentment and confusion. They don't understand that she's barely had time to go to the bathroom, let alone take a shower or have a nap. It is exhausting to have total responsibility for someone twenty-four hours a day with no time to yourself. It is also exhausting to work outside the home all day and then be handed a baby to take care of as soon as you walk in the door. Both parents need time to rest and recuperate.

I have had mothers tell me that they moved into the nursery with the baby so that their partner's sleep wouldn't be disturbed during the night. It's commonly accepted that the man's rest and well-being must be protected because he has to get up and go to work the next day. Unfortunately, a woman who protects her partner in this way will not get the rest she needs.

❧

GABRIELLA WAS AN orthopedic resident's wife who was struggling with postpartum depression. Her husband, Joe, had managed to find someone to cover for him at the hospital when his wife was delivering the baby, but he'd had to return to work immediately after the baby was born. He was on call every third night, which meant that he had to spend the night in the hospital to cover any emergencies. Because he was almost finished with his training, however, he got to sleep through most of the night while the younger residents did most of the work. He was called only when a situation became too complicated.

Gabriella was convinced that because Joe worked during the day, it was her job to take care of the baby at night. After all, she wasn't "working," and he needed his sleep so that he could get up for work the next day. Joe wasn't insisting on this arrangement, but Gabriella thought it was fair, and Joe didn't volunteer to give up any sleep.

Gabriella's mistake was assuming that she wasn't working. In many ways, she was working harder than Joe, and she was certainly getting less sleep. She never got more than two or three hours of uninterrupted sleep and was either breastfeeding or attending to the baby when she was awake. She frequently didn't shower or get dressed until Joe came home, and then she took only half an hour to get cleaned up. She was running on empty and about to break.

Gabriella and Joe came to see me when she confessed that she was having thoughts of death and imagining who would take care of the baby when she was gone. When she described their parenting arrangement, I said, "You can't keep going like this. Joe is going to have to help you. You are both Claire's parents, and you both need to share the burden."

"I'm more than happy to get up with the baby, but Gabriella insists on doing it all herself," Joe replied. "I feel totally left out, like they have something special going on and I'm not welcome. I know Gabby's tired. I don't know how she's done it. But I want to feel like I'm part of the deal. I should be tired, too. It's our baby."

I wanted to make sure Gabriella heard him. "Gabriella, did you hear what he was saying? You are very lucky to have a husband who wants to contribute. Joe is willing to get up with the baby."

She was very quiet, then said, "I just wanted to make it easier for him. He works so hard, and I didn't want his life to be disrupted."

I laughed. "There is absolutely no way that either of your lives is not going to be disrupted. Your lives are now officially disrupted forever. But you can only survive parenthood as a team. It hasn't happened to just one of you. Your child needs both of you.

"Joe, if Gabriella is breastfeeding, you could get up with the baby and hand her to Gabriella to nurse. Then when the baby is finished eating, you could change her diaper and put her back to bed." Joe nodded. That didn't seem to be too much for him at all. "Keep the baby in your room in a bassinet while she's waking up so frequently. You want to make everything as easy as possible when you have to get up at three in the morning."

Then I turned to Gabriella. "I just can't stress enough how important it is for you to get some uninterrupted sleep. It would be okay to substitute a bottle for one of the nighttime feeds so that you could get at least four or five hours of sleep in a row. It will make a big difference in how you feel."

Gabriella and Joe agreed to share nighttime baby duty. With medication, therapy, and some sleep, she was able to recover from her depression.

Gabriella was one of millions of women who find themselves cast into a depression after having a baby. But she was lucky to have the good sense to get some help when she needed it. Other women don't descend into actual depression, but they are wracked with guilt over their ambivalence about becoming parents. The first three months of a baby's life serve as a strong reality check for people who have dreamed of becoming parents but don't have the foggiest notion of what that involves. Of course, having a child enriches one's life immeasurably, but it's critical that both parents go through a period of adjustment.

※

BEYOND THE NEED for parents to care for their new baby together, there is the need to stay emotionally and physically close to each other. This includes sexual intimacy. For most couples, sex is how they ended up with a baby in the first place, and with luck sex will resume after the woman has healed physically. Sexuality is an important part of most intimate relationships. It connects couples emotionally and can often be a way to close the distance and repair hurt feelings, which are part of the landscape for two people trying to parent together.

Most physicians recommend waiting six weeks after the birth of a child before resuming sexual intercourse. For some couples, this can seem like an eternity. For others, reconnecting sexually is terrifying. Both partners may be apprehensive about the woman's changed body and may wonder whether sex will still be enjoyable for them.

Resuming sexual activity after giving birth can be daunting. Both the man and the woman may be afraid that it will be painful for the woman. Whether she had a vaginal delivery or a C-section, she needs to heal. Going slowly and not expecting the sexual experience of a lifetime can help. Sex can be difficult to discuss at any time, let alone when you are struggling with being a new parent. But talking helps, as does having a sense of humor.

Breastfeeding can complicate the reconnection process. Estrogen levels remain low when a woman is breastfeeding, and this can cause a decrease in sexual desire and vaginal lubrication. Many women report that even though they can think about enjoying intimacy with their husbands, they experience no physical response or a greatly decreased response to stimulation. Until breastfeeding is over and hormone levels return to normal, this lack of response interferes with a normal sex life. Using a lubricant can help, and patience and understanding by both partners can get the couple through some less than sexually fulfilling moments.

Women also often complain of feeling overwhelmed by their intense physical contact with the baby. At the end of the day, the thought of having anyone else "on them" is intolerable. Sex is the last thing on many new mothers' minds. And many fathers struggle with feeling left out and ignored. Mom spends so much time and energy with the baby that it feels as if she has nothing left for her partner. The tension between these two positions can cause great frustration for both parents.

In addition, it's hard to experience sexual desire when you are sleep deprived. After being awakened steadily throughout the night, sleep is the only thing you want. When the baby is sleeping, it is a magical time, and sex certainly might break the spell. It's hard to think of anything except the sleeping baby and how not to wake him up. And it's difficult for anyone to enjoy sex while listening for a baby.

You may have trouble seeing yourself as both a mother or father and a sexual being. None of us likes to equate sexuality with parenting. Who wants to imagine his or her parents having sex? And then all of a sudden, *you* are the parents. For this reason, it may be hard to think of your partner (and yourself) in a sexual way.

The most important thing is to make time for your partner. Don't forget that your marriage needs to be the primary relationship. Marriages are hard to sustain in the best of circumstances, but many couples make the mistake of focusing all their attention on the baby and forgetting that they need care and attention, too. Too many marriages fall apart because the parents spend so much time caring for their children that they lose touch with each other.

Schedule time to be alone with your partner. A newborn can tolerate one hour away from his or her parents. Go for coffee; if you're breastfeeding, make it decaffeinated. When family members come to visit, ask if they will baby-sit while the two of you take a walk around the block. As soon as possible, spend a night at a hotel. You don't have to go far, just someplace where there is no baby to feed, no crying to wake you up, and no older children in the next room. Remember what it's like to be alone, just the two of you, before there were any children. One day it will be just the two of you again, and it's nice to remind yourselves along the way why you chose each other so many years ago.

Returning to Work

The fourth major adjustment in this fourth trimester is going back to work. Some women feel terrible about leaving the baby; other women feel terrible that they're looking forward to resuming their work life. It's never easy, and there are always sacrifices.

When I was in training to become a psychiatrist, the surgical residents worked harder and longer than any others. Whereas I had to take overnight call every four or five days, the surgeons were often in the hospital for thirty-six hours straight every two or three days. It's an exhausting pace. A few residents drop out of the program every year because they are unable or unwilling to tolerate the schedule. The surgeons consider themselves very tough. Taking time off because you are sick, tired, or postpartum is just not an option.

There were only a handful of women training to be surgeons in the early nineties. Women were not considered tough enough to withstand the hardships of the surgery schedule. No concessions were made for any woman who became pregnant during her surgical residency. She had to continue to work, staying up all night every two to three nights, regardless of her protruding belly.

I watched as one of the female surgeons became more and more pregnant. I was amazed at how she continued on without missing a beat. I was struggling with the grueling pace of being an intern, and I wasn't pregnant. As she looked to be getting closer and closer to delivery, I wondered how long she was going to last. One day I noticed she was at work, no longer pregnant. That was confusing because I thought I'd seen her just a week or so before, looking huge. I wondered if something bad had happened and asked her if everything was all right.

"Oh, yeah, it's great. I had a baby boy, and everything's wonderful."

I was now really confused. "How old is he? You were still pregnant just a couple of weeks ago. Did you take any time off from work at all?"

"I was really lucky. I didn't have to come back until he was a week old. It was hard to get someone to cover for me, but I had about four days of vacation and got another three days by trading with people. Fortunately, I was able to work until I went into labor. It worked out pretty well; no one's too mad at me for being gone."

I was incredulous. I wanted to ask her about breastfeeding and who was taking care of the baby and whether it was hard to leave him after only a week. I'd already had one baby, and there was no way I could have gone back to work one week after delivery. I couldn't have done it physically, and I wouldn't have wanted to try. This colleague took it in stride. What choice did she have? If she wanted to be a surgeon and a mother, this was the way she was going to have to do it.

※

I WAS LUCKY to have more choices. I stayed home for varying amounts of time after the birth of my children. I took six weeks off after my first baby was born. That was barely enough time to grasp what had happened. I wasn't ready to go back to work or to leave my baby in the care of someone else. Something profound had happened, and I needed time to absorb it. I was just starting to relax and enjoy being a mother. I did go back to work, but I couldn't think about anything except my baby. It was torture, and I'm sure I wasn't at my best.

After my second child, I took eight weeks off. It was definitely better than six weeks. Amazingly, those two extra weeks made a big difference. It takes six weeks for mother and baby to establish a routine and begin to understand each other. Right when that happens, many women have to return to work and don't get to revel in the feeling of being competent. Returning to work is essentially a crisis; it is a disruption of the schedule you just established.

Returning to work means that you have to figure out who's going to stay with the baby, what time you will have to get up in order to get everything done before you leave the house, what time you will have to leave work so that you can pick up the baby or let the nanny go home. Just when things were getting better, your whole world is turned upside down again. If you continue to breastfeed, you have to make sure the baby will take a bottle, have breast milk stored, and figure out where and when you're going to pump at work. I have used a breast pump in some pretty strange places, with my foot wedged up against the door so that no one could come in.

With my third and fourth children, I took a full three months off. Heaven. By the time they were three months old, they had made a place for themselves in the family. There was a clear routine, and we were all comfortable with the new addition. I also felt totally connected to them. I knew their language, what their cries meant, and how to respond. They were also sleeping longer at night, and I could get at least four or five hours without having to wake up to feed them. It is such a glorious moment when your baby sleeps almost all night. Waking up every two or three hours to feed your baby can take a terrible toll on your moods, especially if you're juggling home and work responsibilities.

Some women decide to stay home even longer — six months or a year — and some choose not to go back to work at all. All of these decisions are right for different women. We need to give mothers permission to do what is best for them and their families. There is no one "right" amount of time to stay home with a new baby, but I think that our society puts too much pressure on women to return to work much too soon after the birth of a child. Six weeks is the absolute minimum, but I believe that three months should be the norm.

The United States ranks at the bottom of the list of industrialized countries in regard to maternity leave. There have been attempts to improve this situation. The Family and Medical Leave Act (FMLA) was passed in 1993 to ensure that workers could take time off following the birth or adoption of a child. The law requires that a mother or father be given up to twelve weeks off and that he or she may return to the same job or a job of similar pay and benefits. Although this is a tremendous improvement over having leave regulated by each employer, the leave is generally unpaid and may be economically unfeasible for a mother or father to take.

Many industrialized countries have had much more favorable leave policies for decades. Sweden, for example, allows up to eighteen months of paid leave at 80 percent of the worker's salary. Contributions by both employer and employee pay for this leave. Swedish citizens pay high taxes, which is not all good, but at least this policy allows families to make mother and infant health and development a priority. Many other countries recognize the importance of parents spending adequate time with their children in the early stages of their lives.

※

THE PHYSICAL AND emotional work of the second half of the fourth trimester takes more than a few weeks to master, but toward the end of this time, baby and parents are beginning to establish a routine, the marriage is starting to show signs of new life, and a joyful family relationship that will last a lifetime is taking shape. Although some women may make it look easy, the truth is that it's a difficult journey to adjust to the physical and mental changes of having a baby and to find your own new normal.

· TIPS ·

1. *Good enough.* There are enough pressures on moms and newborns from the outside; women don't need to put additional pressure on themselves. Allow yourself to be good enough, and don't expect perfection. Although some women make it look easy, you never know what is going on inside someone else's home. I see "perfect" families in my office every day that are actually in shambles when you get up close.

Find other mothers to talk to. Pick the woman in your child's playgroup with spit-up stains on her shirt. She probably will be happy to listen to your frustrations and fears — and to share hers with you.

Don't listen to advice about the "right" way to do things. There are many right ways, depending on whom you ask or what books you read. Some tell you to sleep with your child; others say that is the worst thing you could do. Most children do fine regardless of where they sleep, although for the sake of the parents' mental health, I am an advocate of having children sleep in their own beds. Pick a method that feels right to you and your partner, and feel confident that you know what is best for your family. Find a pediatrician with whom you feel comfortable and stick with his or her advice. Even pediatricians disagree on issues as important as feeding newborns and deciding where they should sleep. Don't judge your situation based on what your sister's pediatrician said.

You won't scar your child for life if you make a mistake. Despite how fragile-looking children are, they are really very sturdy. Aside from neglect and child abuse, it is hard to do anything to a baby that will damage him or her irreparably. Using or not using a pacifier will not make any difference in the long run. Wearing designer clothes or eating gourmet organic baby food will not result in a healthier, happier child. Taking time to love your child, play with him, and read to him *will* make a difference, and the abundance of good things that you do will far outweigh any mistakes that you make.

2. *One night a week.* Your relationship with your partner has to come first. Your child will be better served by having the example of parents who love and care for each other than by having parents who make her the center of their universe. Relationships often falter as the stress of raising a child overwhelms the tenuous intimacy of husband and wife.

Spend one night a week alone, without your child. It doesn't have to be elaborate or expensive. Find a sitter, walk to the nearest park, sit on a bench, and talk. Get a cup of coffee or take a drive in the country. Do anything that gets you out of the house, away from your child, and focused on each other. If you're anxious about leaving your newborn, you don't have to be gone long. Just an hour can be enough to help the two of you feel connected.

For the duration of your marriage, try to get away occasionally for at least one overnight while a friend or relative watches the kids. It may be as simple as spending the night at the Holiday Inn down the street. Being able to watch a movie uninterrupted or have sex without worrying about hearing the sound of tiny feet padding down the hallway is a luxury for couples with small children and can help sustain you through some pretty chaotic times.

Every day, take half an hour for yourselves. This can be at the beginning of the evening before supper or after the kids are in bed. Use this time to talk about your day or what's coming up for the week ahead, or to check in on each other's emotional health. Pick a time when you will not be interrupted and you're not too tired to pay attention. As your children grow, they will see two parents who love and respect each other and are committed to making their marriage work.

3. *The best of both worlds.* Going back to work can be an emotionally painful time for a new mother. Even if you're looking forward to returning to work, it's hard to leave your sweet-smelling newborn behind.

For the baby's safety and your mental health, it is imperative to find childcare that you trust. You can't concentrate on work if you are anxious about how your baby is doing with the sitter or at the daycare center. You need to feel that your child isn't lacking for nurturing or comfort while you are away.

Most women who are successful at combining work and motherhood learn how to compartmentalize. This means that when you are at work, you are focusing on work and not trying to take care of things at home. At the end of the workday, you leave work behind and focus on your family. Don't bring work home unless there are extraordinary circumstances. Don't try to play with your child while composing memos on your laptop.

You won't be doing either job well, and your child will be unhappy not to have your undivided attention. Nobody wins in those situations.

For some women, working part-time is the best of both worlds. For others, part-time work or staying home is not a financial option. Whichever situation works for your family, the most important issue is to make sure that your child is well cared for. That care could be provided by a nanny, a daycare worker, the father, or another relative, but it must be loving care by a consistent caregiver. Your child will know you are Mommy even if you're not there every minute of the day.

8

When More Help Is Needed

Nora brought her newborn home from the hospital with great fanfare. Baby Elizabeth was much anticipated, and the whole family was on pins and needles until she was born and safely home. On Nora's first day home, she got into bed for a nap and put Elizabeth in the bassinet beside her. She was exhausted; hospitals are not easy places to sleep.

Then the phone began to ring with good wishes. Nora answered the first few calls but then asked her mother to run interference. She settled back down to sleep. After only fifteen minutes, Elizabeth woke up crying. Nora started to undo her nightgown to breastfeed when the next-door neighbors knocked on the door to see the baby. The whole family trooped in, oblivious to the fact that Nora was half-clothed. After half an hour of arguing over whose turn it was to hold the baby, they finally left. Nora tried to start nursing again. Her mother interrupted to inform her that she had invited an old friend and her family to dinner.

"You what?" Nora exclaimed. "I can't believe it. I'm having company for dinner?"

"Don't worry, honey," her mother said. "I'll cook, and you don't have to do anything. They wanted to see the baby, and I just couldn't say no. It'll be fine."

Nora took a deep breath and decided that she could stay in her bedroom and hide. Once again, as she was trying to get Elizabeth to nurse, the doorbell rang. It was her brother. Nora lost it. She started screaming for everyone to get out of her house.

"My mother came running to try to calm me down, but by that point I was sobbing hysterically," she told me. "It was all just more than I could handle. My poor brother. An hour later, I was feeling better, and I was embarrassed at how out of control I was. But it was all so hard, and I was so tired. I just wanted to get in bed with the baby, feed her, and sleep. Why don't people realize how hard it is to have company the day you bring the baby home?"

Baby Blues

Nora was in my office at the insistence of her mother. The family was worried that something was seriously wrong and wanted to do whatever they could to help. Nora's baby was ten days old, and she had brought Elizabeth with her. While Nora was talking to me, she held Elizabeth and gently rocked the baby in her arms. She frequently looked down at Elizabeth and adjusted her daughter's blankets. She spoke to me quietly, hoping that Elizabeth would stay asleep.

I asked Nora if she was getting enough sleep.

"Oh, my gosh," she said. "I could sleep all the time. I'm so tired, the minute I lay my head on the pillow, I'm asleep. The next thing I know, it's time to feed her again."

"Are you enjoying being a new mom?"

She immediately grinned and said, "It's great. Don't get me

wrong, it's really hard, and there are some days that nothing seems to go right, but already I can't imagine my world without Elizabeth. But I don't know what's wrong with me. I'm so irritable with my mom. I know she's trying to help, but if she invites one more of her friends over while I'm trying to breastfeed, I think I'm going to crack. I just wish I didn't cry so much. Do I have postpartum depression? I don't feel depressed. I feel really happy about having Elizabeth."

After asking her several more questions, I assured her that what she was experiencing was not depression, but something called the baby blues. The baby blues affect up to 80 percent of all women who deliver a baby. The symptoms are not severe and do not impair a woman's ability to care for herself or her baby. The blues come on about three days after delivery and should go away by two weeks postpartum. A mother may feel tearful, irritable, and anxious about her responsibilities as a mother. She may complain of moodiness and break into tears for no reason. But she also experiences periods of pleasure and enjoys her new baby. Her appetite is good, and she is able to sleep when the baby sleeps. As a matter of fact, she is desperate for sleep and falls asleep easily.

Pregnancy and the postpartum period are times of extreme hormonal variation for all women. Estrogen and progesterone levels rise throughout pregnancy. By the end of pregnancy, the levels of these hormones are hundreds of times higher than before the woman became pregnant. Then the baby is delivered, and quickly thereafter the placenta. The placenta has been responsible for secreting large amounts of these hormones. Once it is separated from the mother's blood supply, her hormone levels begin to drop precipitously. In most women, this rapid decline causes the baby blues, but in a small group of women, these changes trigger frank depression (see the next section).

Baby blues symptoms are similar to the premenstrual symptoms that many women experience. One of the most frightening things about the baby blues is that many women don't expect them and aren't sure what is happening or why. If a new mother isn't aware that she is likely to experience the temporary but tumultuous baby blues, she may be frightened by them. Women are told by television, books, and other mothers that giving birth is one of the most fulfilling things they can do. If the bonding process is interrupted by the baby blues, they add to the woman's fear that she won't be a good mother.

One of my friends recently had a baby. I visited her when her son, Jonathan, was six weeks old. We were sitting in the living room while she nursed. Everything was going well for her; she was enjoying her time off from work and was having fun caring for her baby boy. I asked her if she'd had any trouble adjusting to motherhood during the first few weeks.

"Not really," she said. "It all went pretty well. My mom and sister came the first week and helped me figure out how to take care of Jonathan. I'd barely held a baby before. Just putting a T-shirt on him was an adventure. I was so afraid I was going to hurt him.

"What was hard was everybody telling me how excited I must be and how wonderful it all was. It wasn't really. I kept thinking, 'I don't feel excited. I just feel tired and sore.' I could barely sit down, and my nipples were cracked from breastfeeding. And then I was crying at the stupidest things — like a dog food commercial on TV or when my neighbor showed up with a spaghetti casserole. I kept hoping it was going to get better, because if this is what having a baby is all about, I didn't ever want to do that again. And then one day, I woke up and it was better. Somehow it all seemed to be falling into place, and I wasn't so emotional anymore. I just wish someone had told me it was going to be like that. I wouldn't have been so worried that maybe there was something wrong with me."

The first few weeks of being a new mother can be overwhelming. Your body is recovering, you are trying to learn how to care for your baby, and you are functioning on very little sleep. One moment you are totally in love with being a mother, and the next moment it all seems too much. Later, looking back on those early weeks, you'll be able to laugh at yourself. But at the time, it doesn't seem at all funny.

Postpartum Depression

Sometimes there is something more serious going on than the baby blues. This is known as postpartum depression. It may be frightening or uncomfortable for a woman to talk about postpartum depression, but keeping silent about this real and treatable disorder will prevent her from getting the help she needs.

It is estimated that 19 million Americans experience a depressive episode each year. Many will go undiagnosed and untreated, often at great cost to themselves, their families, and their employers. Women are much more likely than men to have depression. Twelve percent of women in the United States, or approximately 12 million women, become depressed every year. One woman in four will experience some type of depression in her lifetime. Think of yourself and your three best friends. At least one of you will likely develop depression at some point in your life. Women owe it to themselves and their families to understand this illness and to demand the appropriate treatment for it.

Postpartum depression is similar to the baby blues but more serious. A conservative estimate is that postpartum depression affects one out of ten women. I believe that it is one of the most underrecognized, underreported, and undertreated illnesses that affect women.

Symptoms of Postpartum Depression

The symptoms of postpartum depression are similar to those of a general depression, but there are subtle differences. Decreased or increased appetite, frequent crying, depressed mood, sleep disturbance, feelings of hopelessness and worthlessness, decreased energy, decreased concentration, and sometimes suicidal thoughts can all be symptoms of depression. Women with postpartum depression may have all of these symptoms, but sleep disturbance is the hallmark of the disorder. Women with postpartum depression cannot sleep no matter how desperately tired they are.

Most women with new babies long for sleep. Getting up every two or three hours to feed a baby is exhausting. After a couple of days, sleeping becomes a priority. You feel as if you could fall asleep just about anywhere. I once fell asleep nursing and dreamed about sleeping!

But women with postpartum depression can't fall asleep, no matter how hard they try. They simply can't turn off their thoughts. One woman described it to me like this: "There's this movie playing over and over in my head, and I can't get it to stop. It never ends, just keeps going and going."

Often these thoughts are worries about the baby. Is he gaining enough weight? Do I have enough milk? Will I be a good mother? Every new mother has these thoughts at one time or another, but women with postpartum depression can't stop them. And the less sleep they get, the more difficult it is to cope with the normal worries, fears, and trials of having a newborn. At some point, they may feel as if they're losing their minds.

In my experience, the single best question to ask a new mother who I suspect is suffering from postpartum depression is, "Are you able to sleep when the baby is sleeping?" Sleep deprivation may be a trigger for postpartum depression. At the very least, lack of sleep worsens depression, and getting enough sleep is a very important part of treating the illness. For some women, two or three nights of uninterrupted sleep can make a tremendous difference in the way they feel and may eliminate the need for antidepressant or antianxiety medication.

❦

I RECEIVED A phone message from a woman saying that her daughter Shelly had been referred to me by her obstetrician and it was important that I see her as soon as possible. I called back and asked what was going on. Shelly's mother told me that her daughter was having panic attacks and was crying all the time. The panic attacks were becoming more and more frequent, and the family was thinking they'd have to take her to the emergency room. Fortunately, I had a cancellation that day and told the mother to bring Shelly in.

Shelly began by telling me that she was having a hard time adjusting to motherhood. She was so anxious about having a new baby and not having any idea what to do. The baby had spit up in the hospital and choked. Although she had handled the situation correctly, she was terrified that something else would happen and she wouldn't know how to deal with it. Her mother was going back to Iowa soon, and the closer her departure date came, the more panicky Shelly felt. She also was crying more and more frequently and was having a hard time getting out of bed in the morning.

I asked Shelly more about her symptoms. She was having

problems with both anxiety and depression. She wasn't suicidal or having thoughts of harming her baby, but she was feeling so anxious that she couldn't sleep at night. She began to cry when she told me how much she and her husband, Benjamin, had wanted this baby and that now she was wondering what in the world they'd done.

"I can't believe I'm telling you this, but I keep thinking this was all a big mistake," she said. "We shouldn't have had a baby. My life was really good before I had Lily, but this is awful. And I feel so guilty for having those feelings." Benjamin was sitting on the couch next to her. I watched his reaction to gauge how he was feeling about what Shelly had just said. I asked him, "How does it make you feel to hear Shelly say those things?"

He very sweetly said, "I'm worried about her. I know how much she wanted this baby, and I feel so bad for her. I keep watching her suffer, and there's nothing I can do to help. I tell her she's going to be a really good mother, but she doesn't believe me for more than ten minutes." He looked at her and smiled.

I talked to both of them about treatment. I discussed medication and how selective serotonin reuptake inhibitors (SSRIs) can be used to treat anxiety and depression. Shelly wasn't breastfeeding, so that wasn't an issue. She and Benjamin seemed open to the idea of taking medication if it was going to help. But I was less certain about starting Shelly on an antidepressant.

"I'm really stuck in the middle about starting you on medicine," I said. They both looked up in surprise. "Your baby is only seven days old. It's really stressful to be a brand-new mother with a brand-new baby. You also had a bad scare when the baby choked. Now you're waiting for something else bad to happen. You haven't gotten much sleep since you delivered. I'm going to recommend that you get at least four to six hours of uninterrupted sleep for the next two nights. Can Benjamin or your mom feed the baby during the night?"

"Sure," Benjamin said eagerly. I think he would have been willing to do anything to make things better for Shelly.

"I'm going to write a prescription for an antianxiety agent and an antidepressant," I said. "The antianxiety agent you can take immediately if you start to feel you're having a panic attack. The medicine will start working in ten to fifteen minutes.

"But I want you to hold off on taking the antidepressant for a few days. Your baby is so new that I wonder if some time and some sleep might make a big difference. I'll give you some medicine to help you sleep at night. You need to have the baby sleep in another room with someone else so that you won't worry about listening for her. I really want you to sleep. Call me in three days and let me know how you're doing."

I got a phone call from Shelly three days later. She was a different person. "I feel so much better," she said. "I slept for eight hours straight last night. My mom and Ben have been great. I haven't had to take any of those anxiety pills since the day I saw you. Everything feels so different now that I've slept some."

Even I was amazed at what a difference sleep made in Shelly's case. I insist that every new mother suffering from anxiety and depression get more sleep, but I have never seen it have so great an effect. It reminded me how important it is to recommend adequate sleep as a treatment. It's so important that I often argue about this with new moms, and I tell them they don't have an option; someone has to come and help for a few days. Hiring a baby nurse or doula is one alternative. Although this is expensive, it is money very well spent.

I checked in with Shelly a few weeks later. She and Lily had adjusted to their life together, and Shelly felt competent to handle anything. Unfortunately, it doesn't always turn out so well. Women with severe depression need medication to help them get better. Sleep can help, but it doesn't always fix the problem.

A Plan for Women at Risk for Postpartum Depression

Some women are at increased risk for developing postpartum depression. If they can be identified when they are pregnant, measures can be taken to prevent depression from occurring or to make sure the symptoms are caught early and appropriate treatment can begin. This can help minimize suffering for both the mother and her family.

Eighty percent of women experience the baby blues, and 10 percent of new mothers will have postpartum depression. This subset of women who develop depression seems to be particularly vulnerable to the hormonal changes that occur during the reproductive years at menstruation, childbirth, and menopause. All women experience these hormonal changes, but only this group responds to these changes by becoming depressed.

The following conditions may signal that you or someone you love is at increased risk for developing a postpartum psychiatric disorder.

1. Previous episode of depression at some time in your life
2. Depressive symptoms during the third trimester of pregnancy
3. Previous episode of postpartum depression
4. Family history of bipolar disorder
5. Severe premenstrual syndrome
6. Poor marital support

The good news is that if women recognize these risk factors and educate themselves about postpartum disorders, they will have a much better chance of ensuring that they and the women around them get the help they need before and after delivery.

One of the more pleasurable aspects of my job is helping a woman who has had a previous episode of postpartum depression to have a more successful experience with her next child. For many women, the thought of having postpartum depression again stops them from having more children. Women who have had one episode of postpartum depression have a 50 to 70 percent chance of having another episode with a subsequent pregnancy. It may not happen with each pregnancy, but the odds are high that it will. Happily, I can recommend some strategies that can prevent or minimize the effects of this difficult illness.

❧

MELANIE HAD EXPERIENCED postpartum depression after the birth of her first child. She'd struggled for the first three months of her baby's life until she called her obstetrician to tell him something was terribly wrong. "I didn't know what was happening to me," she told me later. "My mom and sister told me it was just the baby blues. They'd all had it, and it was no big deal. But this didn't seem to get better the way they said it would. I was just sinking deeper and deeper into a pit. I don't even remember a lot of that time; I was just going through the motions. I can recall taking care of the baby, but nothing pleasurable about that time at all. By the time I saw my doctor, I was pretty desperate."

Melanie was in my office, two months' pregnant with her second child and terrified that she would become depressed again. Her current obstetrician was a colleague with whom I collaborate closely, and he knew to send her to me before she delivered. It is important to have a plan in place before the delivery so that everyone knows what to expect and what will happen if something goes wrong. It is much easier to try to prevent an illness than to play catch-up after it happens.

After Melanie's first child was born, she responded well to a combination of sleep, medication, and psychotherapy. After four or five weeks, she felt like her old self again. But now she felt that she had missed a really important time with her baby. "I didn't get to do any of the stuff I imagined," she said. "I don't remember his first bath or first smile or any of the sweet times. Once I was better, it was as if I woke up and had this four- or five-month-old baby that I had to get to know. I missed out on so much. I don't want to lose that time again."

Melanie and I talked about her options. She had stayed on medication until her baby was a year old and then tapered off. He was now three years old. I told her, "You have done really well for the past several years and currently don't have any symptoms of depression. It doesn't make sense to start you on medication right now, because you don't need it. I have found that many women who get postpartum depression will start having symptoms in the months right before delivery. After the baby is born, the symptoms can become as bad as the ones you described having. So one thing we will do is to keep a close eye on you while you're pregnant to make sure you keep doing well. I'll want to see you every couple of months or so."

"Okay, I can do that," she replied. "It's comforting to know that you'll be watching me, too. I think last time, I was feeling really bad before I noticed that something was going on. I try to act as if everything's fine most of the time. I don't like to complain."

"Having depression is not the same thing as complaining," I

said. "I want you to notice if you start not feeling well while you're pregnant. If so, we'll talk about it. Some of what you experience may be normal complaints related to being pregnant. We'll try to sort those out from what may be depressive symptoms. One recommendation I'd like to make is that we plan now to put you back on an antidepressant about four or five weeks before you're due to deliver. That way, you will have time to get the medication in your system, which we hope will prevent another episode of depression."

Melanie wanted to know if she could wait and see if she needed to take medicine.

"Some women choose to wait to begin medication, until they see whether they start feeling bad after the delivery. There is always a chance you won't become ill again and you won't need medication. It's important to know, though, that a recent study found that for women with a history of postpartum depression, starting them on an antidepressant prior to delivery prevented another episode. I think it's a decision you will have to make for yourself. But given how bad you felt last time, I think it would be reasonable to try to prevent it from happening again. In my practice, that has worked well for most women.

"Whether you take medication or not, I will want to see you more frequently in the month or two before you deliver. I would like to meet with you and your husband several weeks before the baby is due to talk about how we will communicate once the baby is born and what to watch out for after you get home. If all goes well, I'd like to see you and the baby two weeks after you deliver, just to make sure things stay on track. You have a good chance of everything going very well, and if you do get depressed again, we can catch it early this time. You deserve to be able to enjoy your newborn."

Melanie felt reassured by the fact that she had made a connection with me and that we had a plan in place to get her through this important time in her life. She wasn't sure yet what she was going to do about taking medication prophylactically, but she was willing to consider it and would keep her appointments with me throughout her pregnancy and after.

❦

SOMETIMES I SEE women who are afraid to get pregnant because of a history of depression requiring medication. Jessica and her husband, Jerry, were referred to me by the psychiatrist who had been treating Jessica for depression for several years. She was thirty-five years old, and they had been married for three years. They felt that it was time to start a family even though they were worried about Jessica's depression and whether she would be able to take care of a baby. Would the stress be too much for her? What if her depression returned? What about postpartum depression? She was especially worried that she wouldn't have the energy or stability to care for a baby if she became depressed.

Jessica's psychiatrist was not familiar with the effects of her medications on a pregnancy and would not be comfortable treating her if she became pregnant. Jessica had called several psychiatrists in town, but either they weren't taking new patients or they didn't want to treat a pregnant woman. She was at the end of her rope when she called me for an appointment. She was convinced that she wouldn't be able to have a baby or that she would have to do it without medication.

I asked her while we were on the phone, "What medication are you currently taking?"

"Well, I've been on Zoloft, trazodone, and Klonopin," she said. "I've been doing really well, but I'm worried about what will happen if you tell me I have to stop them."

"Why don't we cross that bridge when we come to it. I'll want to ask you questions about your psychiatric history and what happens when you are off medication. Then we'll talk about the particular drugs and come up with some options. Will your husband be able to come?"

"Does he need to be there?"

"If he can, I think it's really important that he comes. This will be a decision that both of you need to make. Please feel free to bring anyone else who may play an important role in your decision making."

"I'll talk to my husband and maybe my mom. I'll call you back to make an appointment when it's convenient for all of us."

"Are things going okay for you?" I asked. "You're not having any difficulties right now? Do you think this is something that can wait?"

"Oh, sure," she said. "I'm fine. We're not in any hurry. We're just starting this process and want to know what is the best thing for me to do about my medication."

I hung up the phone and smiled. Jessica and Jerry were planning ahead, and I would have time to help them make good decisions.

When Jessica called to schedule an appointment for her and Jerry to see me, I asked if she wanted to talk to me by herself first. She said no, they'd like to come in.

Some women like to schedule an appointment by themselves first. Sometimes a woman wants to tell me something that she's uncomfortable talking about in front of her partner. If a woman asks to see me alone first, it may signal that there is some disagreement about the pregnancy or difficulty in the marriage.

All women need to be screened for possible domestic abuse. Surprisingly, the risk of domestic violence increases during pregnancy. Although the reason for this is not clear, sometimes when a person is at his or her most vulnerable, he or she is a target for another person's aggression. A pregnant woman cannot easily defend herself and is very concerned about the safety of her unborn child. An abusive partner is struggling with his own insecurities, and beating up on her in this especially vulnerable state can make him feel even more powerful.

Jessica and Jerry clearly had no abuse issues, and I was able to walk them through all the options without any of us feeling as though we had to act quickly. We made another appointment to talk further, so that they could be sure to make the best decision for them.

Postpartum Psychosis

Fortunately, postpartum psychosis is extremely rare, but it is also extremely frightening. Postpartum psychosis is a true psychiatric emergency. It is one of the few psychiatric illnesses that scare me. I chose to go into psychiatry because I enjoyed the work and the patients, but also because it was a specialty that allowed me to have some control over my schedule. There are very few times when I have to get up at night or work on the weekends. Postpartum psychosis is an exception. I will drop whatever I am doing, morning, noon, or night, to deal with someone who is experiencing this problem.

To be psychotic means that a person is having hallucinations or delusions, or that the person's thoughts are disorganized and illogical. Hallucinations can be auditory, visual, or tactile, and they occur in the absence of any stimuli. The person believes that he or she is actually hearing, seeing, or tasting something that is not really there.

A delusion is a fixed, false belief. Despite evidence to the contrary, the person is certain that it is the truth. A delusion can be bizarre or non-bizarre. An example of a non-bizarre delusion is a neighbor who believes that you have trained your dog to use only his yard to relieve herself. No matter how hard you try to convince your neighbor that you are an equal-opportunity pet owner, he is convinced otherwise. This is a delusion because you have not trained your dog in this way. You could take pictures of your dog relieving herself in another yard, and your neighbor would claim that the pictures were staged. It is a *non-bizarre* delusion because it is possible but not true.

An example of a bizarre delusion would be a person who believes that the CIA invaded his home at night and removed all of his internal organs. Obviously, if all of your organs were removed, you would be dead. But you cannot convince the delusional person that it's not true. If I were to show him an x-ray of his lungs with his name on it, he would tell me, "That isn't my x-ray. The CIA switched it."

Delusions are extremely hard to treat. Antipsychotic medication can be helpful, but the delusions often remain firmly entrenched.

Mothers who have postpartum psychosis sometimes hear voices in their heads telling them to harm themselves or their babies. These voices are often religious in nature. It is not uncommon for a psychotic woman to have delusions about the baby and to believe that her baby is possessed by the devil or is in danger and must be sacrificed in order to protect him. This is why postpartum psychosis is so dangerous. What seems impossible to you and me seems real to someone who is psychotic.

How is it possible to believe that something is real when it seems so obviously impossible? Different areas of the brain are activated when we think, move, or receive sensory input. When someone is hallucinating or delusional, the relevant areas of the brain "light up" even though the normal input or stimulus is absent. It is impossible for hallucinating people to know that what they are thinking, seeing, or feeling is being generated by their brains without any external input. Brain scans show that when someone is hearing voices, certain areas of the brain are working just as if the person were really hearing someone speak.

Women who have delusions about their children need to see a psychiatrist immediately and usually require hospitalization. Postpartum psychosis can occur in women who have no history of mental illness. About half of these women will be diagnosed with bipolar disorder, or manic-depressive illness. Women with previously diagnosed psychotic illnesses, such as schizophrenia or bipolar disorder, have up to a 50 percent chance of becoming psychotic after delivery. These women need to be closely monitored after childbirth, and if their medication was stopped during the pregnancy, it needs to be restarted immediately.

No one knows what causes postpartum psychosis, but it is believed that the hormonal shifts that occur after delivery are a trigger. Postpartum psychosis can happen very quickly, sometimes within three days of delivery. The illness often begins with agitation and restlessness, then progresses to hallucinations and delusions. It is possible that the sleep deprivation that accompanies new motherhood may contribute to the development of psychosis.

Fortunately, postpartum psychosis occurs in approximately only 1 in 1,000 women. Although postpartum psychosis is rare, it is often tragic if it is not immediately recognized and the mother and her infant are not protected.

I have treated several women with postpartum psychosis, and fortunately all of them have had a good outcome. I am always anxious when treating a woman with this disorder and hold my breath until the delusions and hallucinations end and the woman is back to her normal self. Treating postpartum psychosis involves the whole family and usually requires that the mother be hospitalized and that someone else take care of the baby temporarily. While the mother is ill, she must *never* be left alone with her baby or other children.

Postpartum Obsessive-Compulsive Disorder

All new parents have anxieties and fears. I don't know of any mother or father who hasn't woken up in the middle of the night in a panic wondering if the baby is still breathing. No matter how hard you try to go back to sleep, you can't rest until you get up and feel the baby's warm breath on your hand.

Babies seem so tiny and fragile, and so helpless. It's hard not to think about all of the horrible things that might happen and not to worry that you will do something that will cause irreparable damage. It's normal to be fearful of giving your baby a bath or of dropping her, or to be afraid that she will choke while you are giving her a bottle. It often takes a few weeks to feel confident about taking care of a small newborn.

Mothers with obsessive-compulsive disorder (OCD) have the same fears and worries, but to a degree that is incapacitating. They can't think of anything else and feel as if they really might do the horrible things they are imagining. Their fears become so overwhelming and consuming that they cannot care for their children.

One of the fears of women with postpartum OCD is that they are going crazy — that they will lose control and the horrible thoughts they are having will come true. The thoughts are intrusive, unwanted, and uncomfortable, and they always involve something terrible happening to the baby. Often the thoughts involve the mother doing something to the baby herself. A mother may see, in her head, herself letting go of the baby in the bathtub, or she may have recurrent thoughts of knives or balconies. The thoughts can take various forms but never make sense to the mother. She knows that they are not things she ever wants to do.

It is important to talk about any obsessive-compulsive thoughts and feelings you may be having so that you can get help. Keeping these thoughts to yourself is dangerous for you and your baby. It is uncomfortable to have these thoughts, but OCD is a medical condition that can be treated. With the proper treatment, these thoughts can be controlled, and you can enjoy being with your baby.

Postpartum OCD and postpartum psychosis are not the same disorder. Postpartum OCD is much more common and frequently occurs at the same time as postpartum depression. The following chart may be helpful in understanding the differences between the two disorders.

OBSESSIVE-COMPULSIVE DISORDER	PSYCHOSIS
Thoughts don't make sense.	*Thoughts are part of an illogical story.*
Doesn't want to act on the thoughts.	Believes that she may need to act on the thoughts to fulfill a plan.
Knows the thoughts are her own.	May be hearing voices or feel as if thoughts are being inserted in her head from outside.
Realizes the thoughts are "crazy."	May be unaware that thoughts are unusual or strange.
Caution should be taken, but no known risk of mother acting on intrusive thoughts.	Emergency: risk that mother or infant may be harmed.

In all these cases, finding the right mental health provider is crucial. Try to be as specific as possible about the symptoms you are having. The Internet can be very helpful in this regard. If there is no mental health care provider in your area who specializes in treating postpartum women, you may want to print out an explanation of the disorder that you think you might have and take it with you when you consult with your medical doctor.

Effects of Parental Depression on Children

What are the consequences for the fetus and newborn baby of the mother's untreated mental illness? A pregnant woman with untreated severe depression may be unable to take care of herself. She may lose weight and be incapable of nourishing her baby. She may be unable to get out of bed in the morning or to get to her prenatal visits. The greatest risk may be suicide, which ends not only the mother's life but that of her unborn baby as well.

It would be a huge mistake to assume that it's safer for the mother to tolerate her depression than to expose her baby to medication. Some research suggests that children of depressed mothers have lower IQ scores, exhibit more behavioral problems, and are more likely to suffer from psychiatric disorders. There is also new research on the direct physiological and biological effects of maternal depression on a developing fetus.

In a study published in the *American Journal of Psychiatry* in November 2002, children born to three groups of women were compared. One group of women had taken fluoxetine (Prozac) during pregnancy, one group had taken an older group of antidepressants called tricyclics, and one group had not taken any psychiatric medication. The children were followed over many years to evaluate the effects of these medications on their development.

The researchers found that neither fluoxetine nor tricyclics had any negative impact on language development, IQ scores, or behavior. But maternal depression did have a negative effect on cognitive outcome. Children whose mothers had severe depression during pregnancy and who had episodes of recurrent depression after delivery had significant delays in language development and other cognitive skills. A mother's untreated depression has long-term negative consequences on the future well-being of the infant. These effects were greater than those found for maternal alcohol consumption.

Having seen many new mothers who are depressed, it makes sense to me that a depressed mom is not good for her baby. A depressed mother doesn't hold her baby as often as a mom who isn't depressed, and she doesn't emotionally engage with her baby as frequently. She also doesn't hold the baby up to her face, making eye contact and those lovely cooing noises that babies love.

ONE OF THE clearest cases of maternal depression I've seen fortunately had a good outcome, as the mother was aware that something was terribly wrong and asked for help. Diana was a radiology resident at one of the local medical schools. She and her husband had just had their first baby, and the pregnancy and delivery had gone extremely well. Diana was a very conscientious student and an excellent physician. She read everything she could about her pregnancy and delivery and made sure that she followed her doctor's instructions exactly.

Unfortunately, after the delivery everything started to go

downhill, and no matter what she did or read, she was unable to make it "turn out perfectly." Diana felt that her daughter, not yet on a schedule at three weeks of age, was too fussy. The baby seemed to want to breastfeed every hour and a half and was never satisfied. Diana's nipples were sore, and she was exhausted. She was staying up all night with the baby because she was on maternity leave and her husband was back at work. She felt that since she wasn't "working" at the moment, she should be the one to get up at night.

They had planned it all so well, but it wasn't going as planned. Diana began to have thoughts of throwing her baby against the wall or just getting in her car, taking off, and never coming back. These thoughts made her feel extremely guilty, and she was scared that she wasn't going to be a good mother.

Most new mothers bring their babies with them when they come to see me, either for lack of a babysitter or because they feel the baby is too young to be away from them. Diana walked into my office looking quite gray and carrying her baby in an infant carrier. I smiled at the sight of the little one and looked in the carrier to make admiring comments. I saw a beautiful baby girl who was snug and secure and sound asleep. "You have a beautiful baby," I said quietly. "She looks so peaceful."

"Well, for the moment she's quiet, but she doesn't stay that way for long," Diana replied tersely. With that, she walked over to the couch and sat down. What happened next was all the information I needed to know that Diana and her baby were in serious trouble. When Diana sat down, she placed the baby carrier on the floor approximately three feet away from her, facing out toward the room. The hood of the infant seat was raised so that if Diana looked down at the baby, she couldn't see in.

I had never seen such an obvious lack of interest by a new mother. I could see the baby quite well, but Diana wouldn't be able to tell if she woke up, spit up, or was having any other difficulty. More important, it would be impossible for Diana and her baby to have any intimate contact.

As the baby began to stir and fuss, I became more and more anxious. Diana ignored her daughter and continued on with her story of how terrible she was feeling and how having a baby was nothing like she'd imagined. The baby's crying brought no response, and I finally had to ask if I could pick her up and try to comfort her. As she turned her head to try to nurse from me, I suggested to Diana that the baby was hungry. Diana took the baby from me, opened her shirt, and proceeded to feed her daughter, the whole time barely looking at the infant. I knew that this mother needed treatment quickly, or she and her baby would continue to suffer.

Four weeks later, after starting an antidepressant, Diana and her baby were back in my office smiling and cooing at each other. The change was remarkable and rewarding.

Nonpharmacologic Treatment Options

Psychotherapy should be considered for anyone who is struggling with a psychiatric illness. Whether depression causes stress in other areas of our lives or stress causes depression is an often debated question. What is clear is that biology and environment are linked when considering the causes of depression. Treatment should address both.

For severe depression, medication is absolutely necessary, but the combination of medication and psychotherapy works better than either treatment alone. For mild to moderate depression during pregnancy, psychotherapy should be the first option. As noted earlier, if a pregnant woman doesn't need to take medication, it should be avoided.

Maya was three months' pregnant when her mother died. Although Maya's mother had been ill with cancer for more than a year, it was still devastating to have to say goodbye. She had hoped that her mother might live long enough to see the new baby.

One month after the funeral, Maya was still having trouble sleeping and felt sad all the time. She wasn't concentrating well at work and was having trouble getting her work done. Her husband noticed that on the weekends, she wasn't interested in doing much and cried at the drop of a hat. They both came to see me at the suggestion of her obstetrician.

"It sounds like since your mother died, things have been really tough for you," I said after listening to her story.

"Yeah. It's like I can't get myself up and going again," Maya replied. "My mom and I were so close. I can't imagine having a baby without her. She was so excited when I told her I was pregnant. I don't know how . . ." Maya began to sob. "She was there for all my sisters' babies. I was so looking forward to getting my turn. It seems like I can't get over it. I'm not even looking forward to having the baby anymore."

After asking her many more questions, I concluded that she was grieving and angry but was still able to function at a reasonable level. She was going to work, keeping her prenatal visits, and gaining an appropriate amount of weight. She was not suicidal and desperately wanted to enjoy her pregnancy and her new baby. She was twenty-nine and had never been depressed before, had never seen a psychiatrist or therapist, and had never been treated with any psychiatric medication. I wondered if talking about what she was feeling and working through her anger might help her a lot.

"I'm not sure that at the moment medication is the answer," I said. "I can understand how sad you are and how cheated you're feeling. I know how much you wish your mother could be here and how lousy it is to miss out on having her around. I think what you're feeling is perfectly normal. But I do think you're stuck and need some help trying to deal with all that you're feeling. I recommend coming in and talking with me once a week to try to help you work through the loss of your mom. I think it'll make a big difference."

Maya agreed to start therapy, and we spent the next ten weeks talking about her sadness over the death of her mother and the loss of her dream of having her mom take care of her after the baby was born. Sometimes acknowledging your feelings and allowing yourself really to feel them helps a lot. Maya felt ashamed that she was angry at her mother for dying and felt selfish that she was thinking about all that she had lost.

Often people feel guilty about having thoughts that they believe aren't "nice" or "right." None of us can help the thoughts or feelings we have. It's normal to feel angry and sad, and even to have ugly thoughts about people. It's often not okay to act on those thoughts and feelings, but having them doesn't make you a bad person. Maya was jealous of her sisters, who had been able to enjoy their mother's help when they'd had their children. It wasn't fair that Maya had been cheated of that experience, but life isn't always fair. We have to do the best we can with the hand we are dealt.

Besides acknowledging Maya's right to feel the way she did, we talked about how she could enjoy her new baby without her mother's help. We discussed who else in her family might be available to help her, and she decided to ask her older sister to come when the baby was born. Her sister was thrilled to help out and felt good about filling in for their mom. Maya decided that she would use her mother's maiden name as a middle name for her child, as a way of honoring her mother and including her in the delivery.

Maya began to feel better and was able to incorporate the loss of her mother into her life. She began to be excited again about having a baby. When her daughter was born, she was sad that her mother couldn't be there, but that didn't take away from the joy the family was feeling. Maya thought of her mother often, and she and her sister talked about how much their mom would have enjoyed being there. Maya still cried sometimes when she thought of her mother, but she was not overwhelmed by the tears. Sometimes she even spent a few minutes thinking about her mother on purpose and allowing the tears to fall. It felt good to remember her.

Several studies support the use of psychotherapy in mild to moderate depression during pregnancy. Several different trained professionals — social workers, psychologists, and psychiatrists — can provide psychotherapy. But psychotherapy is becoming less and less a part of psychiatric training. Some psychiatrists today just prescribe medication and refer patients to other practitioners for therapy. I prefer to do both medication management and psychotherapy. I feel fortunate to be able to provide complete treatment for my patients, and it's rewarding to establish close relationships with them. I think doing therapy is a lot more interesting than writing prescriptions.

There are many ways to choose a therapist. The most important factor is that you and your therapist have a good fit. If you meet with someone for the first time and feel uncomfortable with him or her, the therapy will not work. You must have total trust in this person with whom you are going to share your secrets.

9

Where Do We Go from Here?

When I dropped my firstborn, Katie, off for her first year of college, I must admit I cried — a lot. I tried not to, but it felt as if I was throwing my baby to the dingoes. I knew all the reasonable things to feel: She has such a great future ahead of her. She's such a wonderful young woman. But I was feeling every cliché in the book: It was only yesterday that I was holding her in my arms wrapped in a pink blanket. Where did the time go?

Although she and I have a terrific relationship, we are not best friends. Mothers and daughters shouldn't be best friends; there are boundaries between parent and child that should be respected. I don't want to know about her sex life, and I know with certainty that she doesn't want to know anything about mine. Those are topics better left for your best friend. But we do have great respect and affection for each other, and I know we love each other's company. When neither of us is being a pain, we have a great time together.

There are many things I wish for her: a great job, a relationship with someone who treats her with tenderness, and healthy children if she wants them. I wonder what her experience with her husband and her children will be. And I wonder if, by the time she is ready to give birth, there will have been any changes in the way we treat pregnant and postpartum women.

Right now, we have a long way to go. Society as a whole needs to change to better protect women and their children during times of vulnerability. Attitudes need to change regarding women's needs during vulnerable reproductive periods. And information regarding the potential for emotional illness needs to be made readily available to every pregnant and postpartum woman and her family.

Houston suffered as a community when Andrea Yates drowned her five children in June 2001. We were shocked and horrified as the media camped outside her home. We struggled to understand what could cause a mother to kill her children. The story was in the news for months. The city was holding its collective breath until the verdict of guilty was entered. Yates was sentenced and sent to prison; for many, worries were calmed now that a criminal was behind bars and we were once again safe.

In response to the Yates children's deaths, the Mental Health Association of Greater Houston started a fund to help educate the community about women's mental health: the Yates Children Memorial Fund for Women's Mental Health Education. Money has been raised from generous donors, and an advisory committee has been organized to oversee the fund. The mission is to educate families and health care professionals about postpartum illness, to promote research on postpartum psychiatric disorders, and to give women information about resources available to them for treatment.

After having a baby, a woman goes home from the hospital with information about episiotomy care, breastfeeding, infant care, and weight loss. Until recently, however, Houston hospitals did not provide any information about what to expect emotionally after you deliver. There was no mention of the baby blues or postpartum depression. You were instructed to see your baby's pediatrician at two weeks and to schedule a follow-up appointment with your obstetrician at six weeks. No mention was made of emotional difficulties, and no resources were provided should you encounter these problems.

As I travel around the country speaking to obstetricians and nurses about pregnancy and postpartum psychiatric issues, many tell me that they don't provide new mothers with information about psychiatric illness. If a woman complains of emotional symptoms, they are not sure what to tell her. There are often no new-mother support groups run by medical or mental health professionals, and no therapists or psychiatrists specializing in women's psychiatric issues in the area.

If a woman's obstetrician believes that she needs treatment, it may take six to eight weeks to get an appointment with a psychiatrist. An obstetrician may want to treat her but is often uncomfortable with psychiatric symptoms or medication. The average obstetrician has not received any training at all in psychiatric diagnosis or treatment, even though he or she will encounter anxiety and depression every day in a clinical practice.

It is time to make changes. Through the work of the Yates Children Memorial Fund, we now have available to every woman who delivers a baby in the Greater Houston area a brochure describing the symptoms of postpartum psychiatric illness. This brochure has been distributed to local hospitals, ob-gyn offices, and pediatricians' offices. Currently, the brochure has been translated into Spanish and Vietnamese, with plans for several more languages.

On September 1, 2003, House Bill 341 went into effect in Texas. Introduced by Representative Carlos Uresti of the Texas legislature, it was called the Andrea Yates bill. It requires that any health care provider who takes care of a pregnant woman or delivers her baby must give her information about postpartum emotional issues and referral numbers where she may receive help.

The passage of the bill is just the first step in changing the way pregnant and postpartum women are cared for in the state of Texas. To date, however, no money has been allotted to enforce compliance, and many ob-gyns and nurse-midwives aren't even aware of its existence. The bill went into effect without any plan for how referral numbers would be provided. And even if women are given referral numbers, will they have the wherewithal to reach out for help?

Another major problem is that many health care providers don't know enough about pregnancy and postpartum issues. As a result, they may either minimize or misunderstand a woman's feelings and symptoms. Many more health care providers must be educated about postpartum issues in order to provide quality referrals to women.

Education is important, but even when women reach out, it is very difficult for those without financial resources to receive help. Many women without health insurance, including those on Medicaid, have no place to go for mental health care other than the emergency room. They cannot afford even modest mental health fees. In a large city such as Houston, people come from many different cultures and speak many languages, and the mental health services available to some of them are fairly limited. In smaller cities or rural communities, there may not be any mental health providers at all. For all of these reasons, creating a list of viable referrals may be difficult, but doing so would be a big step toward making a positive change.

A local pediatrician recently asked me to speak to his group practice about postpartum depression. Although pediatricians do not take care of mothers directly, it is in their patients' (the babies) best interests to have depression-free mothers. This group of pediatricians has agreed to consider administering the Edinburgh Postnatal Depression Scale (EPDS) to mothers of newborns at the eight-week visit. The EPDS is a self-report questionnaire (see the appendix) that can be filled out quickly by a new mother as an initial screening tool to detect depression. Many of the symptoms of depression about which physicians normally ask patients are normal in a new mother, particularly fatigue and lack of interest in usual activities. The EPDS asks about depressive symptoms that are common in postpartum women. This scale has been found to be reliable and valid in many countries.

A woman typically follows up with her obstetrician six weeks after delivery and then does not return until a year later. This visit typically focuses on wound healing, breastfeeding, and birth control. There is little time to ask sensitive questions about emotions. By contrast, an infant visits the pediatrician at two and eight weeks and at four, six, nine, and twelve months. There are many more opportunities for a woman to be observed with her infant during these visits. As a result, it may be in the pediatrician's office that women with postpartum depression can be more easily identified and given appropriate referrals for evaluation and treatment.

Support Groups

Once a woman has been identified as having depressive symptoms, she needs to find a professional who can help. Houston, a city of 4 million people, has just two postpartum support groups. But Houston isn't out of the ordinary. When I recently asked a large group of obstetricians if they knew of any postpartum support groups in their communities, the answer was a collective no.

Support groups can be an integral part of a new mother's care. Even if she is taking medication for a postpartum illness, medication alone often is not enough. She may need a place to go where she can talk with other mothers who understand just how she's feeling. Both medication and support can be ideal.

A support group typically has two trained leaders who help keep the group on track and make sure everyone gets a chance to express herself. Support groups are wonderful places to talk about thoughts, feelings, fears, and worries without feeling judged. If you say that you think you are the worst mother in the world, someone else will probably say that she felt that way in the beginning, too. One nice thing about a support group is that it may include a wide range of women who are at different phases of their illness. Some will be new mothers, and others will be over the worst of their illness and now living healthy lives with their babies.

I recommend a support group for all of my patients. One of the biggest difficulties with postpartum illness is the sense of shame and guilt. Perhaps you feel as if you're the only one in the world this has ever happened to. As a result, you think that you need to keep it a secret. Having others to talk to who have had similar experiences will help you put your struggles in perspective.

Mother-Infant Units

It is extraordinarily difficult to tell a new mother that she has to leave her home and be admitted to the hospital for postpartum treatment. Not only does it force the woman to leave her baby behind, but family members and friends must scramble to find someone who can temporarily "mother" the infant. If the mother is breastfeeding, the situation is even worse. Although it is possible to get a breast pump in the hospital, it can take a day or more for the pump to finally get to your room.

In Europe, particularly England, some hospitals have mother-infant units where mother and baby can stay together. The nurses in these units are specially trained in mental health care, postpartum care, and infant care. This is a major advance for the treatment of women and their babies. The mother is able to receive the best care for herself, and she does not feel the guilt and anguish of leaving her baby behind. As far as I know, there is only one such unit available in the United States.

Standards of Care

Standards need to be developed to define optimal care for postpartum psychiatric illness. Standards are the minimum level of care provided by health care professionals when treating specific illnesses. They are used to evaluate doctors when there is a question of negligence: was the doctor performing up to the customary standards of care? Physicians aren't required to be perfect, or the best at what they do, but they must adhere to a minimum standard. It is up to each practitioner to make sure he or she practices medicine according to these standards.

Currently, there are no standards for the diagnosis and treatment of postpartum depression. You may or may not receive adequate care from your physician, but this is not necessarily your doctor's fault. Postpartum illnesses are just beginning to be taught in medical schools and training programs. In addition, there is little research available to guide physicians in determining the best course of action in a particular situation. The treatment of postpartum psychiatric disorders is still considered to be best handled by an "expert."

I believe that anyone who cares for pregnant and postpartum women can follow a few simple guidelines.

1. Every woman needs to be given information about postpartum disorders, preferably prior to delivery, so that she knows what to expect and when to ask for help.
2. Women at increased risk for postpartum illness need to be identified before delivery, and a follow-up (by phone or in person) should be scheduled for two weeks postpartum.
3. Every woman should be asked about mood and anxiety symptoms at her first postpartum visit.
4. Any woman with a history of postpartum illness should make contact with a mental health professional prior to delivery.
5. Any woman diagnosed with a postpartum psychiatric illness must be asked about thoughts of harming herself or her baby.

National Changes

Women around the country are suffering from postpartum illnesses. Some well-known women have used their own situations to further the awareness and recognition of these disorders. In 2001, Marie Osmond wrote an account of her struggle with postpartum depression and how she got help. More recently, Brooke Shields wrote a moving account of her depression after the birth of her daughter. She described in detail the feelings and fears she experienced while she first tried to deny the problem and then later sought help. She has become a champion for women's mental health. These and other well-known women have helped to remove the stigma of having a postpartum illness, and now other women may feel less ashamed to ask for help.

In New Jersey, Mary Jo Codey, wife of former governor Richard Codey, disclosed her history of postpartum depression. Her advocacy led to sweeping changes in the state. For example, August 2005 was declared Postpartum Depression Month, and the New Jersey Department of Health and Senior Services funds a program to educate citizens and health care professionals about these issues of women's reproductive mental health.

Slowly, the nation is becoming more aware of the emotional health needs of new mothers and of women in general. Attitudes and expectations about the care and support women need when they are expecting or have just delivered a child are changing.

Conclusion

In 2006, Andrea Yates was retried for the deaths of her five children and found not guilty by reason of insanity. It is my belief that this was a just and merciful verdict for a woman who was suffering from a severe postpartum psychosis and received, in my opinion, inadequate medical help for it. She will more than likely spend the rest of her life in a state psychiatric facility where she can receive competent and compassionate care.

In part because of this case, Americans are more aware of the potential for harm if postpartum symptoms are ignored or misread. As a result, we have an opportunity to make tremendous changes in the way we care for pregnant and postpartum women. Making those changes will benefit not just the mother but also everyone who comes in contact with her, including her child.

Our mothers are integral to our well-being. They give us the sense of ourselves as lovable, good people, no matter how high we rise or how far we fall. Those are feelings we need to carry with us for the rest of our lives in order to survive the normal losses and disappointments that inevitably come our way. Without good mothering (which in some families is done by a father, grandmother, or other primary caretaker), we struggle with feelings of low self-esteem, have difficulty with intimate relationships, and are at increased risk for psychiatric disorders. Without intervention, we will transmit our trauma to our own children.

When a mother I have helped calls to tell me how well she is doing and how much she is enjoying her new baby, I am rewarded by knowing I have had an impact on many lives. Her child will live a healthier and happier life if she is emotionally available to him. Making an intervention early in a mother's life with her child can prevent long-term mental health, educational, and social problems. My good friend Maureen says, "Mothers are the glue that holds society together." If we protect our mothers, we protect ourselves and our futures.

❦

MY DAUGHTER KATIE is graduating from college this year. She says she wants to go to medical school and become a child psychiatrist. I know that she may change her mind, but what a compliment she has paid me just by considering doing what I do. She is proud of me, the work I do, and the things I believe in.

My five-year-old daughter is about to start kindergarten. She reminds me of myself as a child: precocious, willful, and enthusiastic about life. There are many years between her and Katie. My life circumstances are different, my energies are in transition, and my desires have changed. I will be a different mother to my five-year-old than I was to Katie when she was growing up. In some ways, I am a better mother now, though less energetic.

But some things are the same for both of them. They are loved, encouraged, supported, and admired. I have made mistakes and will continue to do so — sometimes the same mistakes over and over again. But I know that I have given them, and will continue to give them, strength and respect for themselves. They will have their own lives to live and their own happiness and mistakes to make. They will know that their mother wasn't perfect. They will know that they, too, only have to be good enough.

APPENDIX

INDEX

Appendix

My Postpartum Plan

The real work begins after the baby arrives. Spend time thinking about how you want those first weeks at home to go. You don't have to stick rigidly to the plan, but thoughtful planning will help reduce your feelings of being overwhelmed by it all.

You can answer some of the following questions well before the ninth month, but others will have to wait until after the baby arrives. You may notice that some of your answers will change as circumstances change.

Who will stay with me?

Week one _____

Arrival date _____

Departure date _____

Week two _____

Arrival date _____

Departure date _____

Week three _____

Arrival date _____

Departure date _____

Dad will take off work from _____ to _____

Who has offered meals?

Week one _____

Week two _____

Week three _____

Resources/telephone numbers for:

Housekeeping _____

_____

Laundry _____

_____

Grocery shopping _____

_____

Baby-sitting _____

_____

Other plans for:

Activities for my other children _____

_____

Comfortable clothes _____

_____

Bedside cooler _____

_____

Who will watch the baby while I'm napping daily? _____

_____

Phone message for first week home _____

_____

Exercise plan _____

_____

When I need a break I can _____

_____

FDA Drug Categories for Use in Pregnancy

CATEGORY	INTERPRETATION
A	Adequate, well-controlled studies in pregnant women have not shown an increased risk of fetal abnormalities to the fetus in any trimester of pregnancy.
B	Animal studies have revealed no evidence of harm to the fetus, however, there are no adequate and well-controlled studies in pregnant women. OR Animal studies have shown an adverse effect, but adequate and well-controlled studies in pregnant women have failed to demonstrate a risk to the fetus in any trimester.
C	Animal studies have shown an adverse effect and there are no adequate and well-controlled studies in pregnant women. OR No animal studies have been conducted and there are no adequate and well-controlled studies in pregnant women.
D	Adequate well-controlled or observational studies in pregnant women have demonstrated a risk to the fetus. However, the benefits of therapy may outweigh the potential risk. For example, the drug may be acceptable if needed in a life-threatening situation or serious disease for which safer drugs cannot be used or are ineffective.
X	Adequate well-controlled or observational studies in animals or pregnant women have demonstrated positive evidence of fetal abnormalities or risks. The use of the product is contraindicated in women who are or may become pregnant.

Source: *Physicians Desk Reference,* 60th ed. (Montvale, NJ: Thomson PDR, 2006).

Examples of Medications Used in Pregnancy

Class A: Thyroid hormone.

Class B: Wellbutrin (bupropion, antidepressant). Although this drug is classified as a Class B drug, there are fewer studies of the effects of this drug during pregnancy than many of the Class C drugs. It is not necessarily safer.

Class C: Prozac (fluoxetine, antidepressant), Zoloft (sertraline, antidepressant), Celexa (citalopram, antidepressant), Lexapro (escitalopram, antidepressant), Effexor (venlafaxine, antidepressant), Cymbalta (duloxetine, antidepressant).

Class D: Paxil (paroxetine, antidepressant), lithium carbonate (mood stabilizer for bipolar disorder). Paxil has been shown to have a small increased risk of a commonly treatable heart defect when taken in the first trimester. Lithium carries an increased risk of Ebstein's anomaly, a more serious heart defect involving the tricuspid valve.

Class X: Thalidomide (anti-miscarriage drug).

Potential Adverse Effects: SSRIs

Neonatal Behavioral Syndrome

Several small studies have indicated that infants born to mothers who take SSRIs (selective serotonin reuptake inhibitors) up to the time of delivery may have symptoms after birth related either to serotonin withdrawal or serotonin overstimulation. These symptoms are relatively mild and are similar to symptoms newborns may have who have not been exposed to serotonin antidepressants. Larger studies have not observed this phenomenon.

These symptoms may include jitteriness or tremulousness,

poor feeding, difficulty maintaining temperature, or hypotonia (or "floppy"). None of the symptoms were severe, and the infants went home from the hospital with their mothers. Some physicians are recommending that mothers taper off SSRIs two weeks prior to delivery. While this may be an option that some parents will want to choose, this puts the mother at increased risk for her depression recurring or for postpartum depression. While the medication may be restarted after delivery, it may be several weeks before the medication becomes effective. As always, the risk to the infant must be weighed against the risk to the mother. These decisions should be carefully discussed with your health care provider. Medication should never be abruptly stopped.

Persistent Pulmonary Hypertension of the Newborn (PPHN)

This is a potentially life-threatening illness that affects blood circulation and oxygenation of the newborn. In one study, published in the *New England Journal of Medicine* in February 2006, there appeared to be a sixfold increase in cases of PPHN in infants exposed to an SSRI after the twentieth week of pregnancy. However, the estimated risk of less than 1 percent in infants exposed in utero is still small and may be less to some women than the risk of untreated severe or recurrent depression. Further investigation is needed to determine the significance of these preliminary results.

Nutritional Supplements and "Natural" Drugs During Pregnancy

I was not taught anything about nutrition in medical school during the late eighties and early nineties. As a future physician, I was taught about disease and pharmacologic treatments. Nutrition was left to the ancillary staff in the hospital who had special training in how to make a balanced meal. As far as we knew, nutritionists helped diabetics with meal planning and helped overweight people lose weight.

Since that time, people have become more interested in the effects of diet and nutritional supplements on their health. Health food stores have proliferated, with aisles full of herbs and vitamins. Alternative medicine — treatments not part of mainstream medical practice — is becoming more and more popular. Many of my patients want to try something "natural" before taking any prescription medication. To them, "natural" means something that can be bought at a health food store or "prescribed" by someone without a medical degree from a traditional medical school. It's important to realize that even something bought at a health food store may still be a drug.

According to *The American Heritage Dictionary of the English Language,* a drug is "a substance used in the diagnosis, treatment, or prevention of a disease." St. John's wort is a plant that is currently being used to treat depression. Although it can be bought at a health food store, it is a drug, ingested in an attempt to treat an illness. Some people believe that because a substance is "natural," it is safer or better than a prescription drug. That isn't necessarily true.

Drugs that I write prescriptions for have been carefully scrutinized in studies with large numbers of subjects and have been approved by the Food and Drug Administration (FDA). Natural substances have not been well studied in carefully designed trials, and the information available about their safety is scarce. While I know the available scientific literature about taking Prozac during pregnancy, there is very little known about the use of St. John's wort during pregnancy. Lithium is a natural salt that was once sold over the counter as a salt substitute for people with hypertension. But lithium has tremendous side effects and can cause heart defects in the fetus if taken during early pregnancy.

Of course, many of the drugs that I prescribe have been derived from substances found in nature. But they are produced by large pharmaceutical companies with strict quality control standards, and they may not be sold to the public until studies prove that the benefits of the drug outweigh any side effects. Occasionally, after a medication has been released to the public, it is discovered to be harmful and is taken off the market. Sometimes it takes several years for a dangerous side effect to become evident. But throughout a prescription drug's life, the FDA continues to monitor and regulate it. A system of checks and balances is in place.

Ephedra is an example of what can happen when a drug is not regulated by the FDA. Ephedra is an herb, commonly derived from the ma huang plant. As a dietary supplement, it is considered a food and not subject to the same scrutiny that the FDA requires for a medication to be made available to the public. Ephedra has commonly been found in weight loss pills and teas. The medication ephedrine is a synthetic derivative of the natural substance ephedra and is used by physicians as a powerful tool to raise blood pressure.

Physicians have known for a long time that weight loss supplements with ephedra were potentially dangerous when taken in excess. I advised all of my patients not to take them. Not only does ephedra increase the risk for stroke and heart attack, but it also can cause depression. Only after many deaths were attributed to these diet pills did the federal government ban the substance. Because ephedra-based substances could be bought in health food stores, many people mistakenly assumed they were safe.

In 1992, the National Institutes of Health (NIH) established the Office of Alternative Medicine with funding of $2 million. Its mission was to study the effects of nontraditional treatments such as yoga, acupuncture, and nutritional supplements. In 1999, the National Center for Complementary and Alternative Medicine was founded as one of the freestanding institutes of the NIH. In 2004, it had a budget of $114.1 million. As more research is being done, "natural" treatments are becoming part of mainstream medicine.

OMEGA-3 FATTY ACIDS

Omega-3 fatty acids are one of the natural substances that have received attention from scientists for several years. Contrary to popular belief, fats are not all bad. In fact, some fats are essential to maintaining good health. These necessary fats are called essential fatty acids, or EFAs. They are essential to good health but can't be manufactured by the body and must instead be obtained through your diet. A diet very low in these fats may actually be harmful to your health.

The EFAs are classified as omega-3 fatty acids or omega-6 fatty acids. (The numbers 3 and 6 refer to the fatty acid molecule and how far from the end of the carbon chain there is a double bond.) Omega-3 fatty acids are found in cold-water fish such as salmon, cod, sardines, herring, and mackerel, as well as in some green leafy vegetables, flax, flaxseed oil, and canola oil. Omega-6 fatty acids are found in many vegetable oils used in the average American diet, particularly corn oil. In addition, much of the meat we eat comes from animals that have been fed diets high in omega-6 fatty acids. As a result, Americans typically consume a diet that has a very high ratio of omega-6 to omega-3 fats.

In 1998, Joseph Hibbeln of the NIH published a letter to the editor in the prestigious British journal *Lancet*. Hibbeln had found a correlation between countries with decreased consumption of fish and depression. Rates of depression were much higher in the United States, for example, than in countries (such as Japan and Finland) where fish is an integral part of the daily diet. He postulated that as humans have changed from the diet of our earliest ancestors, which was high in omega-3 fatty acids (wild game, fish, and grains), to a diet rich in omega-6 fatty acids (processed grains, dairy products, and farm animals), we have become more depressed.

Researchers studying heart health, arthritis, and cancer have found benefits from consuming fish oil, which contains high concentrations of omega-3 fatty acids. Now there is growing interest in investigating fish oil for the treatment of depression, bipolar disorder, schizophrenia, attention deficit disorder, and other psychiatric illnesses. I attended one of the first conferences on the use of fish oil in psychiatric disorders, held at the NIH in April 1999. Researchers from around the world gathered to discuss possible uses for omega-3 fatty acids in psychiatric illness.

Both omega-3 and omega-6 fatty acids are polyunsaturated fats that make up part of the membrane that surrounds each cell in the body. The highest concentrations of omega-3 fatty acids are found in the brain and the eye. Receptor molecules, such as the serotonin receptor, sit in the cell membrane, and it is thought that omega-3 fatty acids provide greater membrane flexibility, enhancing the cell's ability to function optimally. It has been postulated that an imbalance in the ratio of omega-3 fatty acids to omega-6 fatty acids in brain cells may be partly responsible for mental disorders.

There have also been studies documenting low levels of omega-3 fatty acids in the red blood cell membranes of persons with depression and bipolar disorder. In a study published in May 1999 in the *Archives of General Psychiatry,* Andrew Stoll of Harvard Medical School and Lauren Marangell of Baylor College of Medicine showed that patients with bipolar disorder who had their traditional medications supplemented with high doses of fish oil stayed well longer and had a much more stable course. Other studies are under way to confirm these findings.

Interestingly, during pregnancy and breastfeeding, large amounts of omega-3 fatty acids are transferred from mother to baby in order to build the baby's nervous system. As noted previously, there is some evidence that low levels of omega-3 fatty acids are associated with depression. Perhaps supplying the mother with more omega-3 fatty acids during and after pregnancy could reduce the incidence of depression. Yet there are many challenges in studying omega-3 fatty acids in pregnant women, as physicians must of course be extremely cautious when recommending any treatment during pregnancy. It is unclear how many milligrams of fish oil would need to be consumed in order to be useful in preventing depression. It also is difficult to know how long it takes for fatty acids to be incorporated into the cell membrane and thus how long before delivery treatment should start. More interventional trials will need to be done to answer these questions.

Another potentially promising area may be the use of omega-3 fatty acids to treat bipolar disorder, or manic-depressive illness, during pregnancy. The drugs used to treat this disorder are very problematic. Lithium can cause a serious heart defect, and other drugs can cause neural tube defects, or failure of the spinal column to close. If there was a treatment for bipolar disorder during pregnancy that was safe and beneficial for the mother and fetus, it would be revolutionary. Studies of using omega-3 fatty acids in this regard are ongoing.

I have had several patients who have chosen to stop taking conventional mood stabilizers because they did not want to risk harming their babies. For women with serious manic-depressive illness, it is not currently the standard of care to recommend stopping medication. But when a woman makes this decision on her own, I recommend that she take fish oil in an effort to prevent a recurrence of her illness, though with the understanding that we are not sure whether fish oil supplements are helpful. Several of my patients have done well with fish oil and have been able to stay off other medications during the pregnancy, but this course should be taken only in close consultation with a physician.

Fish oil is extremely safe. It has been studied in pregnant women in Sweden as a treatment for pregnancy-induced hypertension. Although it did not prove to be effective in treating this disorder, there were no adverse outcomes in any of the women or their babies due to the fish oil. The most frequently reported side effects are stomach upset and "fish burp." Fortunately, several companies now make flavored capsules that eliminate the latter problem.

A theoretical and more serious side effect is the risk of increased bleeding due to the metabolic effects of omega-3 fatty acids. Studies looking at this problem have found no increase in bleeding time in patients, and in the studies of pregnant women in Sweden, no increased bleeding was noted after delivery. Although fish oil may be useful in heart disease because it reduces the "stickiness" of platelets (one of the body's tools to clot blood), it does not seem to increase the risk of bleeding in individuals taking it as a supplement.

If fish oil is taken during pregnancy, it is important to find a pharmaceutical-grade product. It will say this on the label. This means that the fish oil has been processed and does not have any other substances in it, particularly mercury. As has been recently discovered, fish may be more contaminated with mercury than we previously thought. It has been recommended that pregnant women consume limited amounts of certain fish. (Mercury causes serious problems for a developing fetus.) Also to be avoided during pregnancy are any fish oil preparations with vitamin A added. Large doses of vitamin A can cause birth defects.

Omega-3 fatty acids are good for both mother and baby. There is some evidence that infants born to mothers who have supplemented with fish oil during pregnancy have better visual acuity and cognitive function at birth. In premature infants, these fatty acids are added to formula to enhance their eye and brain development. More and more over-the-counter formulas contain these fatty acids as they become recognized as essential building blocks for growing infants.

I suggest fish oil as a potential tool for many of the pregnant women I treat. Although there is not yet any conclusive research proving that it is safe to use in place of conventional treatments, there's also no evidence that it is harmful when taken as a dietary supplement during pregnancy.

Edinburgh Postnatal Depression Scale (EPDS)

The EPDS was developed as a tool to screen for depression in women at the 6- to 8-week postpartum visit. This short, self-report tool can be administered in a clinical setting or in a woman's home. Responses are scored 0, 1, 2, or 3 according to the severity of the symptom. The questions marked with an asterisk (*) are reverse scored (i.e., 3, 2, 1, and 0). The total score is determined by adding the scores of each of the ten questions. A score above 13 is considered positive and the woman should be referred for further evaluation. Any indication of suicidal ideation, even if the total score is below 13, and the woman should be referred immediately for follow-up by a health professional. This scale is not intended to replace a complete assessment by a licensed health care professional.

INSTRUCTIONS FOR USERS

1. The mother is asked to underline 1 of 4 possible responses that comes the closest to how she has been feeling the previous 7 days.
2. All 10 items must be completed.
3. Care should be taken to avoid the possibility of the mother discussing her answers with others.
4. The mother should complete the scale herself, unless she has limited English or has difficulty with reading.

Name: Date:
Address: Baby's Age:

As you have recently had a baby, we would like to know how you are feeling. Please UNDERLINE the answer which comes closest to how you have felt IN THE PAST 7 DAYS, not just how you feel today.

Here is an example, already completed.

I have felt happy:
Yes, all the time
<u>Yes, most of the time</u>
No, not very often
No, not at all

This would mean: "I have felt happy most of the time" during the past week. Please complete the other questions in the same way.

In the past 7 days:

1. I have been able to laugh and see the funny side of things:

As much as I always could
Not quite so much now
Definitely not so much now
Not at all

2. I have looked forward with enjoyment to things:

As much as I ever did
Rather less than I used to
Definitely less than I used to
Hardly at all

*3. I have blamed myself unnecessarily when things went wrong:

Yes, most of the time
Yes, some of the time
Not very often
No, never

4. I have been anxious or worried for no good reason:

  No, not at all
  Hardly ever
  Yes, sometimes
  Yes, very often

*5. I have felt scared or panicky for no very good reason:

  Yes, quite a lot
  Yes, sometimes
  No, not much
  No, not at all

*6. Things have been getting on top of me:

  Yes, most of the time I haven't been able to cope at all
  Yes, sometimes I haven't been coping as well as usual
  No, most of the time I have coped quite well
  No, I have been coping as well as ever

*7. I have been so unhappy that I have had difficulty sleeping:

  Yes, most of the time
  Yes, sometimes
  Not very often
  No, not at all

*8. I have felt sad or miserable:

  Yes, most of the time
  Yes, quite often
  Not very often
  No, not at all

*9. I have been so unhappy that I have been crying:

Yes, most of the time
Yes, quite often
Only occasionally
No, never

*10. The thought of harming myself has occurred to me:

Yes, quite often
Sometimes
Hardly ever
Never

Source: J. L. Cox, J. M. Holden, and R. Sagovsky, "Detection of Postnatal Depression: Development of the 10-item Edinburgh Postnatal Depression Scale," *British Journal of Psychiatry* (1987): 150, 782–86.

Postpartum Symptoms Checklist

The Yates Children Memorial Fund for Women's Mental Health Education (YCMF) was created by the Mental Health Association of Greater Houston in June 2002 to provide information and education about postpartum illness to women and their families, as well as to health care providers and others.

Created in memory of Andrea Yates's children — Noah, John, Paul, Luke, and Mary — the YCMF has developed a brochure, *Your Emotions After Delivery,* which has been distributed throughout Texas and other communities in the United States. This brochure includes a postpartum symptoms checklist in English, Spanish, and Vietnamese about postpartum psychiatric illnesses, along with appropriate referral sources.

The YCMF also has sponsored community education events and training for health professionals in the diagnosis and treatment of postpartum depression. A Web-based training course is available, and a certificate of completion will be given upon taking a ten-item posttest.

The Postpartum Symptoms Checklist is meant to help new mothers identify postpartum symptoms — for themselves and their health care providers.

After your baby is born, you may feel:
- Joyful
- Nervous
- Excited
- Worried

These are normal feelings. Many women have them. Some women have more upsetting feelings such as:
- Extreme fear and worry
- Great sadness
- Not feeling normal

Keep reading to learn more about the feelings you may have after having a baby.

Baby Blues

As many as 8 out of 10 new mothers have the "Baby Blues." Signs include:
- Crying
- Mood swings

- Having a short temper
- Being very sensitive

This is similar to what women experience before their periods. The signs start about three days after having a baby. They go away on their own in about two weeks. A woman with "Baby Blues" can still enjoy being a new mother.

POSTPARTUM DEPRESSION

This is a common illness in new mothers. It occurs in 1 out of 10 women after having a baby. Signs may include:

- Sadness
- Having a short temper
- Crying
- Problems sleeping, even when the baby is sleeping
- Not wanting to hold or touch the baby (not enjoying the baby)
- Feeling tired
- Changes in eating patterns
- Thoughts about her own death or the death of her baby

POSTPARTUM ANXIETY

It is normal for new mothers to worry about their babies. But worry that takes over your life is not good for you or your baby. Signs that a mother may be worrying too much are when she is:

- Afraid that something will harm her baby
- Afraid that she will hurt her baby
- Afraid to be alone with her baby
- Spending most of her time trying to get these ideas out of her head or trying to protect her baby

Postpartum Psychosis

This is an illness that happens to 1 out of 1,000 women having a baby. It is an emergency. A mother may:
- Become confused
- Be nervous or very quiet
- Hear voices
- See things
- Have thoughts about hurting herself or her baby

Symptom Checklist

Please check all that apply to you:
- I feel worried or afraid a lot.
- I have not been able to think clearly.
- I am afraid to be alone with my baby.
- I feel cut off from the world or like I do not know what is real anymore.
- I have trouble sleeping even when my baby is sleeping.
- I have not been taking good care of myself (not eating or sleeping).
- I do not enjoy being with my baby.
- I do not want to get out of bed.
- I do not want to be around my friends or family.
- I have had thoughts about death or killing myself.

What Can You Do to Feel Better?

If you are having any of the feelings listed above, please talk to your friends, family, or doctor. If you are afraid you may harm your baby, call your doctor or clinic or go to an emergency room right away. Help is available. You are not alone. Many women feel like you do. Your life will get better when you get help.

Resources

American Psychiatric Association
1000 Wilson Blvd., Suite 1825
Arlington, VA 22209-3901
www.psych.org

National Institute of Mental Health
6001 Executive Blvd.
Room 8184, MSC 9663
Bethesda, MD 20892-9663
www.nimh.nih.gov

Emory University Women's Mental Health Program
Emory University School of Medicine
Emory Clinic Building B
1365 Clifton Road NE, Suite 6100
Atlanta, GA 30322
www.emorywomensprogram.org

MGH Center for Women's Mental Health
Massachusetts General Hospital
Simches Research Building
185 Cambridge Street
Boston, MA 02114
www.womensmentalhealth.org

Depression After Delivery, Inc.
www.depressionafterdelivery.com

Postpartum Support International
927 N. Kellogg Avenue
Santa Barbara, CA 93111
www.postpartum.net

Mental Health Association of Greater Houston
Women's Mental Health Initiative (YCMF)
2211 Norfolk, Suite 810
Houston, TX 77098
www.mhahouston.org

Index